interventions that will inspire and equip anyone working in this challenging yet rewarding field. Comprehensive in its scope, this book leaves no aspect uncovered. It is essential reading for every service and practitioner, encouraging deep reflection on the crucial role each person plays in the journey of trauma recovery.'

*– Lynn Miller Child, Protection Review Manager and Trauma and Promise Champion, Aberdeenshire Council*

'I can't reiterate enough how inspiring and empowering this handbook will be. The clear explanations make it accessible to parents, carers and professionals alike and bring an overwhelming feeling of hope and the possibility of recovering from trauma. I look forward to being able to share this handbook with colleagues and friends who are supporting others through trauma and trauma recovery.'

*– Tracey Dudgeon, Advanced Pupil Support Worker, West Lothian Council*

*of related interest*

**Child Trauma and Attachment in Common
Sense and Doodles – Second Edition**
**A Practical Guide**
*Dr Miriam Silver*
*Illustrated by Teg Lansdell*
*Foreword by Kim S. Golding*
ISBN 978 1 83997 912 5
eISBN 978 1 83997 913 2

**The Complete Guide to Therapeutic Parenting**
**A Helpful Guide to the Theory, Research and What it Means for Everyday Life**
*Jane Mitchell and Sarah Naish*
ISBN 978 1 78775 376 1
eISBN 978 1 78775 377 8
Audio ISBN 978 1 52936 518 4

**The Adverse Childhood Experiences Card Deck**
**Tools to Open Conversations, Identify Support and
Promote Resilience with Adolescents and Adults**
*Dr Warren Larkin*
*Illustrated by Jon Dorsett*
ISBN 978 1 83997 142 6

**The Trauma Treasure Deck**
**A Creative Tool for Assessments, Interventions, and Learning for
Work with Adversity and Stress in Children and Adults**
*Dr Karen Treisman*
*Illustrated by Richy K. Chandler*
ISBN 978 1 83997 137 2

'A must-read and essential text on trauma by a true expert. This book takes readers on a journey well away from all-too-common stigmatizing and over-diagnostic narratives, to one which helps us see children for who they are, for what they really need, why they act as they do and, most importantly, how we can spot genuine trauma in children and help them recover. De Thierry writes with an easy style and makes her points using a wide range of the most important clinical and neuroscience theories, all worn lightly. Fundamentally, this is that rare thing – a text that genuinely helps professionals, therapists and parents reach into the worlds of traumatized children and help them to actually recover. This book will be a boon to so many who need just this kind of guidance in working with the most traumatized children.'

*– Dr Graham Music*

'Betsy de Thierry's book is an essential read for anyone interested in understanding trauma. It provides a thorough contextual analysis that is not only insightful, but also adaptable to various cultures and contexts. The author's ability to address trauma in such a comprehensive and culturally sensitive manner is truly commendable. This is a must-read for professionals and individuals alike.'

*– Rami Khader, Executive Director of Anar for Empowerment*
*and Psychosocial Support, Bethlehem-Gaza | Palestine*

'I immersed myself in this fascinating book over a series of cross-country train journeys and by the time I reached my final destination I was practically equipped to be a better doctor, friend and parent.

Betsy has the extraordinary capacity to take what the world often labels as chaos or disorder in children and give scientifically credible, clear, logical frameworks and language around what young humans naturally do to adapt to terror, powerlessness and overwhelm in life, and offers practical, realistic, meaningful guidance for the trauma recovery journey.

If we want our children, families and societies to thrive on every level, from the individual to the political and economic realms, trauma recovery for children after experiences of injustice and harm is non-negotiable. Betsy challenges us again to understand trauma differently, to question the accuracy and ethics of current groaning narratives of huge numbers of "disordered" or "misbehaving" children and gives scientifically grounded, coherent, practical, realistic and proven steps to reach that trauma recovery goal.'

– Dr Laura Carolyn Wood, Forensic Paediatrician, Yorkshire

'Betsy de Thierry has drawn on years of clinical and supervisory experience to richly capture some of the elements and underpinnings of supporting children on their trauma recovery journey. The book is written in an accessible, warm and engaging way and speaks to therapists, schools, parents, carers and anyone else working with a child who has experienced traumas. In this book, Betsy focuses on sharing her Trauma Recovery Focused Model ®, which offers readers lots of ideas and guidance, as well as powerful acronyms and vignettes. This is one to not be missed.'

– Dr Karen Treisman

'An absolute must-read for anyone supporting children and young people who have experienced trauma. The thoroughness of this book will support anyone in their desire to enable recovery from trauma.'

– Dr Lisa Cherry

'From the moment I read the very first chapter, I found myself utterly captivated. It is a rare treasure, a profoundly written book that I couldn't put down. Every page resonated with the compassion, knowledge and understanding that are hallmarks of Betsy's work, reflecting a deep sense of empathy, caring and kindness in your understanding of the traumas children endure.

The structure of the book is masterful, with reflective questions at the end of each chapter that provide invaluable opportunities for learning and development. As a practitioner, I found that every question I had was addressed in the subsequent pages, showcasing Betsy's thoroughness and foresight.

This book will undoubtedly become my "Trauma Bible," a cornerstone reference for supporting children and their families on the path to trauma ecovery. In conclusion, this book is much more than a guide; it is a lifeline for practitioners dedicated to trauma recovery. It offers a wealth of wisdom, knowledge, practical advice and empathetic

# THE TRAUMA RECOVERY HANDBOOK

A Model for Navigating Recovery
for Professionals, Parents and Carers

## BETSY DE THIERRY

Illustrated by Sarah Hawkins

Jessica Kingsley Publishers
London and Philadelphia

First published in Great Britain in 2025 by Jessica Kingsley Publishers
An imprint of John Murray Press

1

Copyright © Betsy de Thierry 2025

Front cover image source: Sarah Hawkins.

A CIP catalogue record for this title is available from the
British Library and the Library of Congress

ISBN 978 1 80501 202 3
eISBN 978 1 80501 203 0

Printed and bound in Great Britain by TJ Books Limited

Jessica Kingsley Publishers' policy is to use papers that are natural,
renewable and recyclable products and made from wood grown in
sustainable forests. The logging and manufacturing processes are expected
to conform to the environmental regulations of the country of origin.

Jessica Kingsley Publishers
Carmelite House
50 Victoria Embankment
London EC4Y 0DZ

www.jkp.com

John Murray Press
Part of Hodder & Stoughton Ltd
An Hachette Company

The authorised representative in the EEA is Hachette Ireland,
8 Castlecourt Centre, Dublin 15, D15 XTP3, Ireland (email: mailto:info@hbgi.ie)

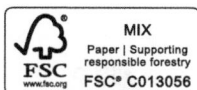

MIX
Paper | Supporting
responsible forestry
FSC
www.fsc.org   FSC® C013056

# Contents

*This book is dedicated to my four sons Josh, Ben, Jonah and Noah, whom I have had the privilege to love, nurture and parent. You are incredible and I am proud of you all. x*

# THE FOUNDATIONS THAT NEED TO BE BUILT

SECTION 1

THE FOUNDATIONS
THAT NEED TO
BE BUILT

# Introduction

I believe that trauma recovery is possible. It's rarely easy and it's rarely fast, but it is possible for children and very much worth the effort. Adults who are survivors and haven't had the opportunity to have trauma recovery support as children may find that the progression to integration and sense of completeness of recovery is more challenging to find, but it is still possible.

In our medicalized system across the world, it is commonplace for the symptoms of human distress to be labelled as a disorder, but I argue that it is often a very ordered way of surviving what shouldn't need to be experienced. People can recover, especially if they are able to understand how they work as a human and what therefore needs to be repaired. I hope this guide will help you and enable you to help many others.

This book is a handbook for professionals, carers, parents and friends who want to do what they can to help someone recover from life-altering traumatic experiences. It is impossible to write a fully comprehensive handbook on trauma recovery – in much the same way that it would be impossible to write a fully comprehensive handbook on recovery from every type of physical injury. There are so many complexities, possible scenarios and individual factors for every specific person's experiences.

## A note on language — primary caregivers and children
The term 'parents' will be mostly used throughout for simplicity, because otherwise the words can be rather lumpy when we use the many different possibilities of primary caregivers such as carers, guardians and other adults.

I also use the word 'child' throughout; this applies to all people aged under 18. However, most of this book is also applicable to adults over 18 who have experienced trauma in their childhood.

## Supporting publications

I have previously written eight 'Simple Guides' which explore subjects that relate to the journey of recovering from trauma. These are:

- *The Simple Guide to Child Trauma*
- *The Simple Guide to Understanding Shame in Children*
- *The Simple Guide to Attachment Difficulties in Children*
- *The Simple Guide to Complex Trauma and Dissociation*
- *The Simple Guide to Sensitive Boys*
- *The Simple Guide to Emotional Neglect*
- *The Simple Guide to Collective Trauma*
- *Teaching the Child on the Trauma Continuum*

This handbook does not aim to replace these, but instead to provide an overview of essential information and good practice to help adults to support, navigate and understand the actual journey of trauma recovery.

You'll notice short extracts from these Simple Guides throughout the book where I think it's useful for the reader to have access to key information. This handbook is self-contained and you do not need to read the Simple Guides in order to use it. For those of you who do wish to carry out further background reading, I have signposted relevant publications at appropriate points.

This book is written for a range of readers, and I'll address each in turn next.

## Welcome psychotherapists, psychologists, creative therapists and counsellors

I am aware that some of you are reading this because you are a qualified and regulated clinical professional working with traumatized children, and you are wanting to make sure that you are fully aware of the different aspects of the trauma recovery journey.

You may be working with a child during school hours all week or supporting children in one-hour sessions per week or leading an after-school group where traumatized children attend, and you are keen to learn how to make sure it is a trauma-informed space where recovery can be facilitated.

This book is written so that you will be able to read and apply some of the knowledge to your important work. It is an introduction to my Trauma Recovery Focused Model® (TRFM®) for trauma recovery focused support. Within this book are 12 of the central tools that have been created for the TRFM®. They are unique to this model and designed over many years whilst working with traumatized families. Please do use them in the way they are designed within the context of the model.

There is a special set of questions for those working as psychotherapists, psychologists and counsellors to help signpost you to additional information at the end of Sections 1 and 2.

In many ways, the content of this book should be known by all professionals who have sought to spend their career committed to helping and supporting children and young people who have experienced the horrors of trauma. I am, however, surprised that the theme of trauma recovery seems to rarely be the focus or priority. I am sure we can all imagine a society that is equipped and intelligently able to carefully intervene and help each child, family and group recover from whatever injustice, pain, turmoil or trauma they have experienced as soon as possible, before any coping mechanisms become normalized for them. I can picture that, and while I recognize the lack of funding and lack of current understanding, this imagined picture of a better world is what is motivating me today to write this book.

## Welcome therapeutic mentors, teachers, teaching assistants, group leaders and other mentors

This book should be helpful for your role, to help you know what you can do and what is not within your role and would be safer for a psychotherapist to facilitate instead. Ideally, each child would have a team around them that would include an adult at home, a mentor in school or another setting and a therapist who can lead the process of recovery and continually assess progression, change, needs and safety. At the end of Sections 1 and 2, there are questions that can help you reflect on your role and aid your development.

## Welcome parents, grandparents, kinship carers and carers

I am aware that some of you reading this book may be reaching out, desperate for some way of navigating the maze of the mental health system, while you are clutching at hope that things could change significantly for that child and family.

You are likely to be reading this to try and equip yourself to fight for the child and for their freedom and recovery. I have also written this book with you in mind, and I hope that it helps strengthen your knowledge and your voice as you seek to support and help. There are questions for you to use to reflect on at the end of each chapter in Sections 1 and 2. I know many professionals who are passionate about working in collaboration with you.

*The book aims to empower everyone involved where often there has been a theme of disempowerment and frustration about the lack of clarity on the process of recovery and healing.*

## What to expect

When I was expecting my first child, I bought a book called *What to Expect When You're Expecting* and I read every page, ticked everything they said I may experience as I went along the journey towards birth, and noted what could come next. I found it a reassuring and helpful aid to a journey that I felt nervous about and for which I wanted to be as prepared as possible. I see this book as a similar handbook to assist and accompany you on the journey of the unknown road, the tough times, when you hope things can change soon. It should lead you to see the child you care for showing positive signs of healing and progression.

I'm hopeful that this book manages to give enough information to equip and empower you to be the kind of helper that every traumatized person needs: an intelligent, caring, empathetic, knowledgeable person who can navigate the maze of different models, methods, theories and solutions. I hope the book is easy to understand and doesn't overwhelm you.

The book will start off exploring the main core foundations that need to be in place for recovery from trauma to happen, and will then look at the primary symptoms and what can help decrease them. It then moves on to explore some specific trauma experiences and what recovery looks like for those.

I want to end this introduction with a note of thanks to the many adults, youth, children and families who have trusted me to support, advise and help them along their journey towards recovery from trauma over the last three decades. I've continued to learn from you.

# CHAPTER 1

# Understanding Trauma

When someone we care about has experienced trauma, and we can see them wrestle with life-altering symptoms, it can feel as if our world is shattered too. We can feel helpless and hopeless, and often the desperation to help and to know what to do can drive us to study and learn. Sadly, there seems to be a distinct lack of coherent exploration or agreement around how trauma recovery can happen or even if it is possible.

I hope this book simplifies the maze of opinion, research and understanding about trauma recovery. I mostly hope that this book brings hope and helps children, young people and indeed adults who were traumatized as a child to begin to recover and find healing and restoration.

The surprise for me over the last decade of training thousands upon thousands of professionals how to facilitate trauma recovery is that currently this topic is not a focus on any qualifying course that I am aware of. Coping with the symptoms of trauma and daily survival seem to be the aim for almost all training courses under the title 'managing symptoms'; I know we can do better.

Research has evidenced that one in three diagnosed mental health conditions in adulthood are known to directly relate to adverse childhood experiences (Kessler *et al.*, 2010). Surely trauma recovery should be the number-one priority across the world to enable communities to flourish and be healthy. I have a dream that trauma recovery could be a central aim for professionals working to support all ages of people, where there is a shared understanding of the impact of trauma and how recovery can happen, with specialist provision that supports those who have experienced trauma and their closest supporters. Otherwise, we may continue to see an increase in devastating statistics of children, young people and adults who are struggling to understand their symptoms and not flourishing and enjoying the gifts and talents that they have. This book aims to give knowledge, which is power, to navigate the systems and enable recovery and help each child to live their full potential.

Gabor Maté (2023), the well-known medical doctor and expert on trauma, addiction, stress and childhood development, asserts that there is good news 'because trauma can be healed. Traumatizing events can never unhappen, but we can heal the wounds they cause' (Shetty, 2023).

Ultimately, I know most of you are keen for a simple step-by-step guide to supporting a specific child or youth through to trauma recovery, and I have aimed to simplify the process while needing to recognize that each child is unique, each trauma story is unique and each child's setting is unique, and as such there is usually a unique path to recovery.

However, there are certainly some clear and essential steps that are necessary for healing. I recognize the sense of powerlessness of waiting for someone to help you, so this book contains as many of the possible elements that are needed to facilitate recovery which are founded in research and decades of practice. The book is aimed at helping parents, carers and primary caregivers to facilitate trauma recovery, as well as being a guide for professionals and organizations to think through the different aspects that are needed to facilitate trauma recovery.

## Trauma

Let us start by looking at what trauma is, so we know what we are dealing with.

Trauma is a word that has become increasingly used. In some ways, this has been helpful and led to some important conversations, changes of culture and further study of the subject, but there has also been a decline in understanding some of the complexities around the experiences of trauma. Many people use the word trauma to describe any event or experience that felt unpleasant in any way, which is a misuse of the term and dilutes its significance. In our society, where so much suffering is a reality, people are finding they need to use words that help their experiences to be validated and evoke empathy, and therefore trauma is often a word used to provoke a reaction of care.

However, I describe trauma in a way that will help us explore the short-term and longer-term impact, so that we can begin to see how we can recover from it. Let's look at some different definitions of trauma.

> Trauma can be defined as any experience or repeated experience where the person feels terrified, powerless and overwhelmed, to the extent that it challenges their capacity to cope. It can leave an imprint on the person's nervous system, emotions, body, behaviours, learning and relationships. (de Thierry, 2021, p.15)

Peter and Levine and Maggie Kline explain trauma and the impact of it succinctly:

> Trauma happens when any experience stuns us like a bolt out of the blue; it overwhelms us, leaving us altered and disconnected from our bodies. Any coping mechanisms we may have had are undermined, and we feel utterly helpless and hopeless. It is as if our legs are knocked out from under us. (Levine & Kline, 2017, p.4)

Gabor Maté explains that:

> trauma is not the event that inflicted the wound. So, the trauma is not the sexual abuse, the trauma is not the war. Trauma is not the abandonment. The trauma is not the inability of your parents to see you for who you were. Trauma is the wound that you sustained as a result. (CBC Radio, 2022)

Some people have lived through so much trauma that they have adjusted to it and their feelings, reactions and behaviours can almost feel normal. They can expect things to go wrong and to be hurt by others and can't imagine a life where things are comfortable. However, they can slowly begin to realize that what has happened to them is unjust and is not an experience of life that everyone shares.

As humans, our response to trauma is a multi-layered system of instinctive, automatic reactions that are in our minds, body, unconscious and relationships. These reactions are the symptoms of distress that haven't been able to be expressed. The symptoms can then become incorporated into the person's everyday life and can seem disconnected from the original experience or series of experiences.

To help facilitate recovery, it is essential that there is an understanding of the overall impact of trauma, and the three words used in my definition – terror, powerlessness and overwhelm – are essential to explore as a foundation.

Remember that trauma can be something that the child experienced *or* something that they didn't experience that they needed *or* both.

So, the trauma we are exploring in this book could be seen as a huge experience or as a smaller, more common experience. Trauma could be a whole range of terrifying experiences where the child is:

- raped, sexually abused or molested
- abandoned or rejected
- teased, mocked or bullied
- ignored, forgotten or neglected
- emotionally neglected
- moved into foster care or residential care
- physically punished or abused
- threatened or intimidated
- controlled by a narcissistic parent
- living in a home with constant violence or arguments
- undergoing a difficult and serious life-altering medical intervention
- misunderstood in ways that cause hurt and shock
- purposefully frightened
- living in a domestic violence or abusive home
- raising their siblings
- experiencing racism
- mediating in conflict between adults
- in a house fire or experiences loss of all possessions
- in a serious car accident
- manipulated to believe or do something they don't want to do
- hungry and without ways to get food or drink
- missing a parent who is away due to conflict, war, prison, separation
- being exploited by an adult or another child
- grieving a sibling or parent or loved one who has died
- looking after their parent emotionally or physically
- looking after a mentally ill parent

- living with parents who have high expectations and use fear to control them
- looking after an unwell sibling
- living in an area that doesn't feel like home
- taking responsibility for things that children shouldn't have to bear the weight of
- unable to experience the constant love and emotional availability of a parent or adult
- moving areas or homes or schools regularly
- being trafficked or exploited by others
- unable to ask for help due to fear or shame
- 'treading on eggshells' due to the home being centred around one adult's needs
- tortured or threatened
- suffering from trauma in the womb or at birth
- stepping up to fill the shoes of a missing parent
- telling lies to keep the family's reputation.

A lot of children who have experienced trauma could be frustrated that they are not able to explain what had happened to them, but they still show the symptoms of distress and dis-ease. Sometimes that is due to them not being aware of a traumatic experience that is buried in the subconscious, sometimes it could be due to preverbal or womb trauma that doesn't have words to describe it, and sometimes they can struggle to use words because it would be emotionally painful and terrifying to speak about it. Gerhardt (2004) discusses the impact of trauma in the womb. She explains that 'as early as pregnancy, the stress response is already forming within the developing foetus and can be affected by the mother's state of health. In particular, her high cortisol level could pass through the placenta into his brain' (p.66).

## Trauma is ultimately an injustice to the soul

It's important to note that while I fully believe that recovery from trauma is possible, we need to know what recovery looks like. Recovery does not mean that you move on from the reality that what happened was unjust, painful, life impacting and a huge disappointment. It is not about forgetting, moving on, being in denial or taking on a victim identity. The concept and journey of recovery will be explored throughout this book, but a brief summary would be that it involves the ability to learn to feel safe, stable, known and validated, while the trauma story is acknowledged and becomes clearer, the impact noticed and the symptoms reduced so that they no longer affect daily life. It is important to note that the stories of the trauma and the recovery should never become over-simplified or ignored, because there needs to be a sense of respect for what has been endured. Herman (2022) explains the core elements of recovery in the context of the core losses: 'the core experiences of psychological trauma are disempowerment and disconnection from others. Recovery therefore is based upon empowerment of the survivor and the creation of new connections' (p.133).

One of the most challenging aspects of the injustice of trauma is the lack of ability to easily speak about what happened, which leads to many people being unable to experience the comfort of relational connection, validation and acknowledgement. This can leave the person feeling that they are invisible and that their suffering and pain are irrelevant to all around them. Worst of all is that perpetrators often know how to manipulate and control the mind of the victims by using techniques to cause the victim to assume they may have exaggerated, made the whole thing up, dreamt it, or they should never tell anyone because more awful things will undoubtedly happen. It can take years and sometimes decades to feel safe enough to even begin to hint at what did occur and then allow themselves to begin to feel the injustice and grief.

## Terror

Terror is described as the feeling of fear that grips your body, mind and emotions. If feeling slightly on edge or unsettled is on one end of the continuum, then terror, which makes your body freeze and your breathing change and time seem to stand still, is on the opposite end. Terror feels threatening to life. Terror has impact that is beyond 'just a feeling' and can automatically grip your body, emotions and mind and cause you to automatically defend yourself to stay alive. The Merriam-Webster Dictionary (2024) describes terror as a word that 'implies the most extreme degree of fear' and is often used with a word that describes the impact of the experience as 'immobilized with terror'.

When someone feels terrified, it isn't actually possible for them to be rational or thoughtful or to just 'get over it' in the same way you can help a child to contain the feelings of anxiety that they may not get an ice cream on a hot summer day because they are at the back of the queue. Terror is an experience that is deeply felt in the body and requires the warmth of relational connection and comfort to process naturally. When other people are not immediately available to provide comfort and reassurance due to the fear of increased terror, or shame or rejection or anger, the person can be left with that feeling inside them for decades. The feeling doesn't leave or dissolve but becomes an unconscious memory that fuels defence mechanisms and reactions without the person knowing why they seem to be 'overreacting' to certain situations.

Terror can cause people to hide, run away, fight or defend themselves because they had to stay alive. Terror can cause people to automatically lose control of their bladder or bowels. People often look back and wonder why they behaved in certain ways and can feel shame or embarrassment about their reactions.

'Now every time I am told that someone is angry with me I have a strong physical reaction that I am going to explode. I have to run to the loo because I seem to lose control of my bladder and bowels in a micro instant. There is no time to reassure myself or calm myself down. My body reacts before I can think of anything.' *Petra, aged 16*

Once someone has experienced terror, it can then cause all other experiences where it is natural to feel a degree of anxiety to be read instinctively as a threat to survival. Little things like children snatching food out of each other's packed lunches can feel terrifying and life threatening to a child who has a history of hunger. They may try and play along for a while, but they may suddenly feel as if they lose control due to the terror of hunger. They may feel shocked and shamed by their reaction and deeply disappointed with themselves because they were so enjoying the friend's company. Their reaction of shouting and being furious, which may have even surprised them, is due to their primitive survival instinct that has been altered due to an early terrifying experience, and now they struggle to differentiate between jokes and real threats. It has been evidenced through a plethora of research that 'children growing up in early adversity are more likely to be emotionally reactive to stress and also less capable of emotional regulation' (Dvir *et al.*, 2014). Therefore, adults need to be able to facilitate help, support and gradual learning around emotions, and this is explored in Chapter 12.

There are many behaviours that are rooted in an automatic reaction to terror that cannot be expressed verbally. Children, youth and adults who have experienced childhood trauma can struggle to use words to express their needs, feelings or fear. They can be as shocked as you may be with their behaviour. Levine (1997) explains that 'words can't accurately convey the anguish that a traumatized person experiences. It has an intensity that defies description' (p.47).

In Sections 2 and 3, we will explore the coping mechanism and defensive behaviours that often develop due to terror. Ultimately, the person needs us to understand that they are reacting to a feeling of terror, and they need comfort, reassurance and our presence to enable them to feel safe from further terror.

### Powerlessness

When a child experiences terror, it can be felt in their body and emotions. The world can seem to stop still. They can feel as if they may die, and they can struggle to breathe as they fight to react to what they are seeing or experiencing. The feeling of terror can be exacerbated because they felt fear due to something that happened or something that they saw or heard happening, and then felt powerless to do anything to stop it. This causes the fear to increase to terror as the child suddenly feels gripped with the reality that they are dependent on adults to care for them. That vulnerability and reliance on adults can feel terrifying when they have not experienced adults to be reliable and nurturing 'enough'. These children feel completely powerless to defend themselves or get out of that situation. The impact of the terror would not be so devastating if they felt they had some power to defend themselves. That is why the younger a child experiences terror without immediate comfort, the more it will negatively impact them through their life. When a child has some sense of power to assert themselves, they can feel less vulnerable to the person or situation that terrified them and so the impact of the trauma is not as deep.

Often a child tries to fight or scream, or they hold those reactions within their body, frozen in time and appearing to be silent and still. This is when they need help to try and express the terror of being powerless in a safe way, to release the trapped energy that is now interrupting their daily life. It isn't that simple, though, and we will explore that further in Sections 2 and 3.

Powerless is both a feeling and a reality for children, and yet when adults empower children to make choices and use their voices to speak up when they need help, then those children don't find themselves feeling terrified about their vulnerability but rather become appreciative of the help from adults. Herman (2022) explains that 'trauma robs the victim of a sense of power and control; the guiding principle of recovery is to restore power and control to the survivor' (p.159).

Powerlessness doesn't have to be terrifying, but when a child is terrified and then finds themselves powerless in the face of the terror, that can be damaging to their perception of the world and how they fit into it.

## Overwhelm

When a child experiences terror and powerlessness, they can develop defence mechanisms and coping strategies that cause them to survive in the short term. What they really need is to be able to process their experiences with an attachment figure with whom they feel emotionally safe. If they are unable to find their attachment figure or if that adult is too busy or seems uninterested, then the child feels further terrified and powerless. The horrific experience of terror has now escalated into a life-changing experience because the child now has urgent feelings and thoughts that need to be explored carefully in order for them to make sense of the world. Without this space to process the experiences with a safe and attuned adult, the child can often begin to show in their behaviour the impact of the feelings of terror, powerlessness and overwhelm.

The impact of feeling overwhelmed is that the child's capacity to 'cope' with all the demands that are placed on them is affected and they react as if they are unable to do much more than find comfort or power. They can struggle to focus on learning things that seem entirely irrelevant to their survival and can easily give up when they are given tasks that challenge them. Their day-to-day life can feel 'overwhelming, unbelievable, and unbearable' (van der Kolk, 2014, p.194).

The child can use the same coping mechanisms as those used by other children who are reacting to terror or powerlessness, but these children often tend to withdraw, be silent or mute and seem content to be in their own worlds where people can't hurt them as much. I usually use the analogy of having internal muddy buckets that 'hold' all the awful things that happen to us. When they get too full, they begin to 'leak', and the overwhelm then becomes apparent externally and people can perceive the overwhelmed child to be naughty or strange.

The word overwhelm describes the need to have emotionally supportive help to 'empty' some of the 'muddy buckets' of emotion, thought and memory in order to feel more able to keep going with the demands of daily life. When someone is overwhelmed, they will sometimes use the words 'I'm just not coping' to describe the feelings that seem just 'too much to carry'. Using the same analogy, a 'golden and shiny bucket' is the place we can hold all our favourite memories to help us have hope and feel less hopeless.

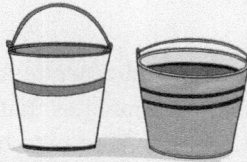

**TRFM® TOOL 1**: The Golden and Muddy Buckets

As the adult supporting a traumatized child, you will also need that space to unpack, process and feel supported and emotionally held by another adult as you navigate the difficult terrain of trauma recovery. It could be that you have support in a partner, friend or a group – even an online group – who understand your journey, because it's tough to do it alone. This is given more time and space in Chapter 9.

'My teachers used to ask why I was groaning in my lessons at school. I didn't know I was groaning, and I didn't know why. I now look back at how traumatized I was due to what was happening to me at home.' *Cara, aged 19*

## The basic neuroscience of trauma

A simplified understanding of the neuroscience around terror, powerlessness and overwhelm is important. When people can understand the automatic, primitive, natural reaction to terror, shame is reduced. When we can explain it to children, they can feel empowered to understand themselves and see that recovery is possible. If we know why we act as we do, we feel more able to change, and this is where simplified neuroscience is important.

We teach children that they have a brain that can be seen as made up of different parts that all have a purpose. A very simple concept is that we have a back brain, which is the brainstem, where our brain's automatic, primitive processes occur from birth. This is also the area of the brain that reacts throughout our life with the automatic fight, flight, freeze response to any possible threat. When that is activated, the thinking brain (prefrontal cortex) is no longer 'working on full power' because the person is trying to stay alive, and this means they have less ability to reflect, think or be reasonable or rational. At the same time as our thinking brain is stuck in panic and freeze mode, and our brainstem is making us react automatically, the limbic area of the brain is also stimulated. The amygdala, which is in the middle of each side (hemisphere) of the brain, begins to alert the body to the danger that is perceived or real, and it causes the people around them to be seen as threatening as the person looks for safety.

When we understand this basic overview of how the brain automatically reacts to threat, we can see the importance of the sequence of what support we offer. For example, we cannot try and have a rational conversation when someone is running away from a place of danger, or if they are screaming in pain. We must first wait for them to feel less terrified, so that they can think and reflect. This may take some time! If a child looks shocked or terrified, we cannot ask them questions about what happened until they feel calmer, because they neurobiologically can struggle to remember anything until they feel safer and less terrified.

Thinking about the brain in terms of two hemispheres can be a helpful way to understand some very simplified concepts about memory and shame. We understand that there is a left and a right hemisphere and our brain stores implicit, non-verbal memory of emotions and experiences in the right hemisphere of the brain. When we can quickly process and make sense of our negative experiences using our left brain, any toxic impact is minimalized. The right hemisphere stores sensory experiences collected and mixed up all together, and the role of the left brain is to sort and file the experiences so that they don't negatively impact our behaviour without cognitive choice and understanding. The brain does that by reflecting, talking, playing and making sense of the experience.

When a child experiences shame, the right brain stores it as a physical sensation and strong emotions. If the shock and fear are too overwhelming, and there isn't a caring, empathetic adult to help process the shock, then the emotions, physical sensations and any accompanying negative thoughts and interpersonal experiences become separated and are stored in the subconscious. (de Thierry, 2019, p.48)

Although the brain stops growing in size by early adolescence, the teenage years are all about fine-tuning how the brain works. Researchers articulate that 'it is well established that the brain undergoes a "rewiring" process that is not complete until approximately 25 years of age' (Arain *et al.*, 2013).

The prefrontal cortex, which is responsible for thinking and being reasonable and rational, is one of the last parts of the brain to mature. This area is responsible for skills like planning, prioritizing and making good decisions. Scientists and researchers are continually discovering more about the brain and how it works, and while this is a very simple overview of the most complex organ of our body, it does help children begin to understand themselves as complex and clever, and enables them to feel less powerless.

## Trauma continuum

To adequately plan the key elements that are necessary to facilitate recovery for someone who has experienced trauma, it is essential to grasp what the impact has been and how multi-faceted it is. In 2015, I first published my theory of The Trauma Continuum, which is a discussion and reflection tool to enable the adults around the child to make sure that there is enough knowledge about the degree of severity of the impact of the trauma experience on the child. It is most certainly not a model for people to compare who has had the hardest trauma or the worst life, but it is aimed at helping facilitate recovery. The Trauma Continuum can help all those who work with children to use a common language, which consequently enables a child to receive an appropriate recovery or treatment plan for their level of traumatic response. The Trauma Continuum is a key element of my TRFM® trauma recovery model:

## THE TRAUMA CONTINUUM

| Type I Trauma | Type II Trauma | Type III Trauma |
| --- | --- | --- |
| Single-incident trauma | Multiple traumas | Multiple pervasive traumas from early age that continue over length of time |

THE TRAUMA CONTINUUM © BETSY DE THIERRY 2015 (DE THIERRY, 2015)

**TRFM® TOOL 2a**: The Trauma Continuum

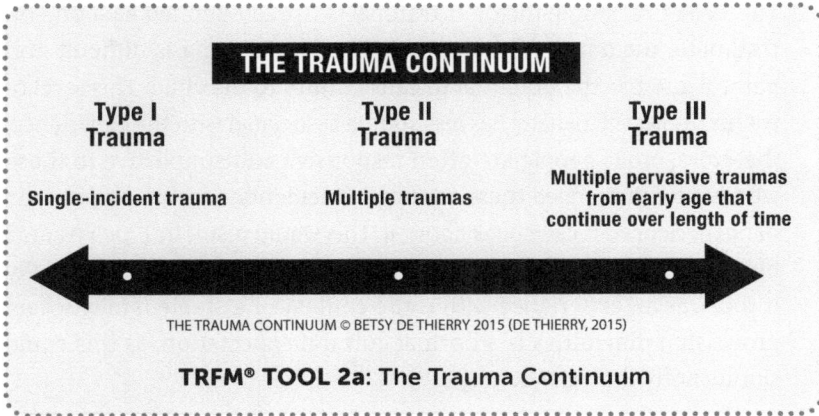

The Trauma Continuum needs to be considered together with The Parenting Capacity Continuum, which illustrates how profound the impact of the traumatic experience may be. It is recognized that the role of parenting is challenging and exhausting, especially when the adults have experienced trauma themselves that still has impact now. Many parents supporting children who are traumatized benefit from investing in their own trauma recovery journey in some way, to help identify their own trauma experience, symptoms and thinking that may be present. While the child needs to be the primary focus of the efforts, it is vital to facilitate time, space and healing for the adult who may need to grieve, identify and then heal from the nurturing relationships they never had, while also providing that for their child. The Parenting Capacity Continuum for the traumatized child is shown below:

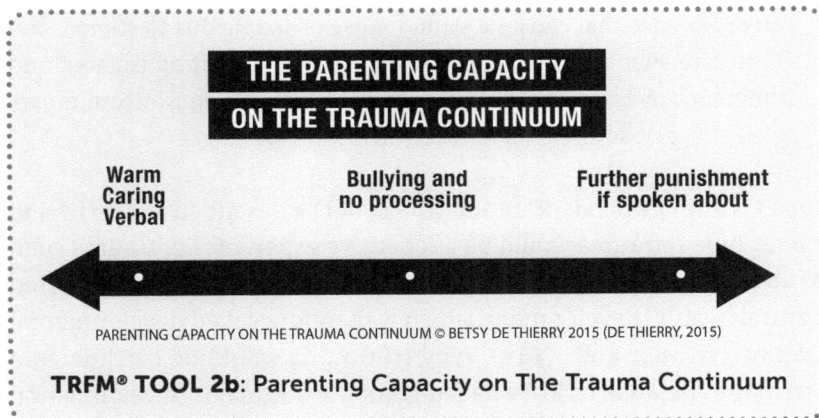

## THE PARENTING CAPACITY
## ON THE TRAUMA CONTINUUM

| Warm Caring Verbal | Bullying and no processing | Further punishment if spoken about |
| --- | --- | --- |

PARENTING CAPACITY ON THE TRAUMA CONTINUUM © BETSY DE THIERRY 2015 (DE THIERRY, 2015)

**TRFM® TOOL 2b**: Parenting Capacity on The Trauma Continuum

The Type I or 'single-incident trauma' is usually defined as a one-off traumatic incident or crisis. Single-incident trauma is difficult and painful and has the potential to cause injury to the child. This level of trauma, however, usually has less stigma associated with the experience; therefore, other people are often responsive and supportive to those who have experienced these traumatic incidents, and the person who has experienced it can speak about it. This would result in Type I trauma being placed at the beginning of the trauma continuum, especially if this was an experience within the context of a stable family where processing difficulties is a normal cultural expectation, as this could significantly limit the damage.

The continuum progresses according to the degree of trauma experienced, the amount of different traumatic experiences and the level of social support and family attachment a child has to enable them to process and recover. Type II trauma involves repetitive experiences that are terrifying; these can rarely be spoken about due to the shock, possible threats, loyalty issues, confusion or a dissociative response due to the level of terror and powerlessness. Type III or complex trauma is positioned at the furthest end of the continuum and involves multiple different traumatic experiences that are serious, repeated and often started at an early age. They could be experiences such as a child who suffers from multiple abuse and/or neglect over many years (pervasive), without a setting in which the traumatic experience could be processed or spoken about in a recovery-focused manner, due to either the primary caregiver's absence, neglect or inability themselves to cope with the trauma. Complex trauma usually involves interpersonal violence, violation or threat and is often longer in duration. It is almost always an experience that causes a strong sense of shame due to stigma, and therefore silence, which can lead to the person feeling isolated and different. For example, repeated sexual abuse, trafficking, torture, organized abuse or severe neglect. (de Thierry, 2015, p.26)

Type I is a single-incident trauma and could be described as a terrifying event. Type II trauma would be a repetitive experience of trauma such as abuse or neglect that has happened in formative years and hindered natural healthy development, which is therefore called developmental trauma (van der Kolk, 2014). Type III trauma would be considered a terrifying life and could be called complex trauma or developmental trauma that varies in the degree of impact depending on other factors that are in the child's life. For example, if a child had a very emotionally present grandparent who was local and nurturing and involved in their life, that would decrease the severity impact of the domestic abuse that they lived in, and so the recovery journey may be shorter. The trauma continuum theory enables the professional to be able to formulate a treatment plan to facilitate the recovery from trauma using information such as:

- What traumatic experiences have been experienced?
- How often did this happen?
- How old was the child when it started? Were they under 5 years old?
- Did the people who should be looking after the child hurt them?
- What are their main trauma symptoms?
- Have they had any other help?

The Trauma Continuum is not a diagnostic tool but an assessment tool to be able to grasp how the trauma is impacting the child, which professional is needed to offer therapeutic support, how long the recovery may take and what trauma symptoms are common for each type of trauma. Without this tool, it is more difficult to work out what may have been causing the symptoms which are life altering for the child, and therefore it is harder to facilitate recovery.

This theory enables the professional to create a treatment plan to facilitate the recovery from trauma. Recovery is possible, but it will always start at the point of assessment so that those supporting the child can begin to grasp where the impact lies and how long those coping mechanisms and defence mechanisms have been working hard to protect them.

## Therapists

This term is now used in a wide manner to mean quite different things! When I refer to 'therapists', I mean a professional who is regulated or accredited by a psychotherapy, counselling or psychology training board. They could be an art, music, dance, play, drama therapist or a psychotherapist or a psychologist, but they are trained academically and practically to work with the subconscious and unconscious. This contrasts with other practitioners who may not have the formal foundations of study in these areas, which I assert are essential to help facilitate recovery from complex trauma.

There are many modalities of psychotherapy and counselling, but I agree with Music (2019) that 'perhaps the biggest problem with the evidence-based practice agenda is that, when you drill down, the real evidence for what is effective seems to be less about the treatment modality and more about the quality of the therapeutic relationship' (p.8). Trauma impacts the body, memory, relationships, emotions, mind, subconscious and unconscious. For trauma recovery specialists, the subconscious and unconscious are the areas that need to be the focus in Type II and III trauma. It is therefore essential that the professional is suitably qualified and clinically supervised for that work to reduce the possibility of symptom escalation and destabilization. A therapeutic mentor is a term I have coined for those who study trauma recovery at length but are not able to be the primary lead professionals due to their different training, but who can offer consistent, long-term support that is less restricted in time and role than that of a therapist.

## A trauma-informed approach to trauma recovery

There has been a recent rise in dialogue, training and documentation using the term 'trauma-informed', and this book is building on the foundation of a trauma-informed practice but with the focus on facilitating recovery from the trauma. Trauma-informed cultures and organizations recognize and validate the impact that trauma has and seek to create safer environments for those who have experienced trauma to be able to be included and feel cared for. Sadly, some organizations or professionals who use the term trauma-informed to describe their practice have somewhat over-simplified trauma and its impact and have practices that are in conflict with the understanding that when adults use any form of shame or fear to alter behaviour, they are exacerbating the trauma responses. While there is indeed a celebration of the worldwide spread of the trauma message, which validates many people's pain and symptoms of turmoil, there is also a degree of frustration at the term being used when the words may clash with the practice of some individuals and organizations. Many professionals who define themselves as trauma recovery specialists are often not equipped to facilitate recovery from complex trauma, and especially not within the area of the subconscious and complex dissociation.

I like to say that there is a difference between doing a trauma-informed training course that is like my first-aid course which sits in 'my back pocket' as a tool for an emergency that I hope I don't have to use, and a trauma-informed training which should be like being given a new pair of glasses. The glasses change how you see the world, the humans within it and what we can all do to bring hope, healing and recovery to those around us and to stand up against injustice. It changes our view, approach, culture and systems to be kinder and intentional towards recovery.

While all people and organizations could be trauma informed and trauma sensitive, I would argue that without a specific trauma recovery model such as my TRFM®, which is explored in this book, trauma recovery is rarely achievable. Crisis recovery is possible, which is the essential support that is needed when someone first discloses or asks for help because they are in a crisis. Trauma recovery is different from crisis recovery. Trauma recovery requires more specialized skills that unpick the layers of the impact of trauma that have occurred while the terrifying experiences have been happening and during all the years since, but crisis recovery is vital to offer help in that critical time of help being urgently needed. Without trained professionals offering specialized trauma recovery therapy working alongside trauma-informed practitioners, it is hard to see how the recovery can be fully achieved, especially with complex trauma.

## Questions to reflect on
### For parents/carers/therapeutic mentors

- What trauma type would the child you are supporting probably be? Why?
- What are their main trauma symptoms?
- What are their greatest needs right now?
- What do they do when they feel terror?
- What do they do when they feel powerless?
- What do they do when they feel overwhelmed?

**For therapists**

- What trauma definition have you been using and why?
- What additional preparations do you make for a child who has experienced Type III trauma compared to one who has experienced Type II?

# CHAPTER 2

# Understanding Normal Human Behaviour

To understand the impact of trauma on the child, we need to understand a little bit about what is perceived as normal behaviour and emotional expression for different ages and stages of a child's life. There are a lot of studies into child development over many decades and it 'is not a unified field, with a single integrated set of theories, nor does one theory or set of theories predominate' (Spodek & Saracho, 1999). However, it is important to explore what behaviour could be due to trauma and what behaviour is deemed an expected part of age-appropriate development. Saracho (2021) explains that child development theories help adults recognize the common progression through childhood and their capabilities at each age and stage. She asserts that these observations provide:

> descriptive statements that help researchers and educators identify the children's abilities and developmental norms that are consistent with their age. A norm is simply an average of the children's characteristics, but it is merely an approximation for each child. Children may be the same in many respects, but they also differ from each other in major ways.

These well-established child development theories explain that children are not born able to use the bathroom and write freely, but they learn such skills at an age that would be recognized as within the range of healthy normal development. Without understanding these milestones, we can assume that the child is distressed or not developing well, and then try and either to facilitate the growth or to look for a diagnosis to relieve our worry. Neither of these is helpful.

Currently, we are seeing children growing up thinking that they have 'something wrong with them' because people seem to have forgotten what normal is!

It is entirely normal for children to:

- be angry and have a temper tantrum – they probably don't have 'anger management issues' but are just angry about something or they are distressed
- need to fiddle with things or move around a lot – that's entirely normal for all children; sitting still is not usually their favourite thing to do at all
- not want to 'do work' and prefer to play – they want to work if they are interested in the matter, but often they would rather have fun
- lie or have amazing imaginations, especially if they can avoid being told off
- zone out and look uninterested in their work because they would rather be playing
- prefer to do what they want to do rather than do what an adult is asking them to do
- whine and complain at the thought of hard work
- be fussy about food and what they eat
- avoid looking an adult in the eyes as it feels uncomfortable and too intense
- avoid challenges where they may fail or look stupid
- miss going to the loo or have the odd accident when they get absorbed in play or their work
- struggle to sit still and focus on learning something they aren't interested in
- hate change and want to avoid new experiences unless they have been reassured
- fear sickness or dying
- not want to go to school and prefer to stay in bed
- struggle to find uniform comfortable and prefer to wear clothes they choose.

I hope you get the point! We need to help children know what normal is so that they don't panic and assume they are in some way 'broken'.

It is devastating to hear so many children expressing authentic worries about these types of issues, as if they need urgent help because they are not like other children. We need to be familiar with what researchers have evidenced is 'normal child behaviour' at the different ages and stages of development.

## Child development theories

Child development has been studied and researched for decades. There are various stages of development that children go through, including emotional, physical, cognitive and social development. They grow and change continually, and while each child is unique, and so they develop in their own time and way, there are some common stages of progression that all children go through. Most parents and professionals are aware of the obvious physical developmental stages in the early years, and teachers are taught about the stages of learning development that occur with school-age children. The education system should be based on these stages so that all adults can balance the role of stimulating a child to keep progressing but not stressing them with too much pressure.

For a child to develop naturally and in a healthy way, they are reliant on their primary caregivers to nurture, care and look after them in a way that enables them to grow without experiencing too much stress. Other than the cognitive and physical developmental stages, there will also be natural development in emotional and social relationships. Just as physical development is reliant on having space to move and explore, and cognitive development is dependent on stimulation, so emotional and social relational development is reliant on enough repeated experiences of relationships and emotions where the adults are able to explain, co-regulate, comfort, guide and soothe.

Erikson outlined an order of these natural psychosocial developmental stages and what the role of the parent is to help them occur. In his theory, as explored by Gross (2020), the child has to essentially move through what seems like a conflict or crisis which needs resolving before progression is made to the next stage of development. In our current context, as a result of pressure and stress seeming to increase while relational richness seems to have decreased – due to screens replacing positive community experiences and causing increased isolation and insecurity – many adults are seeking to understand distress through the filter of diagnosis. They ask, 'What is wrong with this child?' rather than, 'I wonder what is happening to this child?' Small crisis, conflict and challenge can be normal experiences within the process of healthy development when the child has strong and positive attachment figures who can help them process the confusion and difficulty.

Erikson sets out the stages and primary activity of each biological age and the 'favourable outcome' and the 'unfavourable outcome'. This can be used as a general overview of the normal development of the child and can therefore enable us to know how to respond appropriately.

When we consider this theory alongside other child development theories, such as those of Freud, Piaget, Skinner and Vygotsky, and become familiar with healthy children and their natural development, we can grasp why we don't generally worry when a child cries at aged 1 when they are picked up by another adult. We recognize that they are naturally and appropriately suspicious of adults that they don't recognize, and they look for reassurance from the faces of their primary caregiver in order to relax in the arms of a stranger. We don't panic when a child who is aged 10 has tests at school and may feel a little sick or anxious or nervous and think they can't do the tests. We know that it's a normal reaction to having tests, but in the context of the child's healthy positive relationships with their adult, they can learn to navigate the feelings of stress and learn what normal reactions to stress feel like and how to manage them. This can form important knowledge and experience that will benefit them for the rest of their life.

We recognize that the child's significant relational influence shifts from being the primary caregivers when they are little, to wider family and social institutions such as schools and clubs as they progress through childhood. Around puberty, the greatest influence often becomes peers and group affiliations. This explains why there is such a vital need to provide healthy group experiences for teenagers as they seek out a sense of identity as part of a group. When we don't recognize this normal developmental need, parents can feel rejected and abandoned by them when they hit that developmental milestone, rather than feel pleased that they are displaying healthy, appropriate development. Trauma interrupts healthy natural development, which is why a trauma assessment explores the behaviours, psychosocial themes and significant relationship issues that are impacted to see what needs to be restored to a healthy developmental growth progression.

## The Window of Tolerance

This is a foundational theory to help us understand when emotions can be appropriate expressions and when they can lead to destabilization or increased distress. The Window of Tolerance enables us to know when to worry and when a child is just being normal and having only short bursts of behaviour and emotional expression that could possibly be concerning. Here is a snippet from my book *The Simple Guide to Complex Trauma and Dissociation* that explains the theory which we will refer to in this book.

> Dan Siegel (in Fosha, Siegel & Solomon, 2009) came up with a theory he called 'the window of tolerance' (p.223), which is used to describe how children who have not experienced trauma can almost always stay within a normal range in their behaviour and emotions, or stay within 'the window'. Siegel describes how when the child has been traumatized, however, they may spend little time within that 'window' and much more time in behaviour and emotions that are either hyperaroused (top of the window) such as aggression, running, fighting, being emotionally reactive, hypervigilant (looking/smelling/listening for the next danger to happen), being agitated and restless. Or they may spend time in hypoaroused behaviours (bottom of the window) where they are dissociative, lethargic, compliant, in a daze, with numbed emotions or inattentive.
>
> All of these behaviours are therefore seen as symptoms of trauma. So rather than looking at these from a medical model (which tends to ask 'what is wrong with them?'), we look at what happened to the child and see that they are reacting to that in a defensive way. So – in the same way that if you put your fingers into a plug socket, your reaction would be one of shock, pain and terror as an electrical current went through you – these behaviours or trauma symptoms are due to the child feeling terror and powerlessness and needing some help from a calm and safe adult to process and make sense of the experiences. When we understand the different reactions to trauma, we can provide calm when the child is hyperaroused and provide activation when the child is hypoaroused. (de Thierry, 2020, pp.45–46)

## HYPERAROUSAL ZONE

**HYPERVIGILANT
FLASHBACKS
EMOTIONAL REACTIVITY
AGITATED AND JUMPY
ALARM RESPONSE**

**WINDOW OF TOLERANCE**

**OPTIMAL AROUSAL ZONE**

## HYPOAROUSAL ZONE

**NUMBING OF EMOTIONS
DISSOCIATIVE
SLOW AND LETHARGIC
GLAZED AND SLOW TO RESPOND
COMPLIANT
INATTENTIVE**

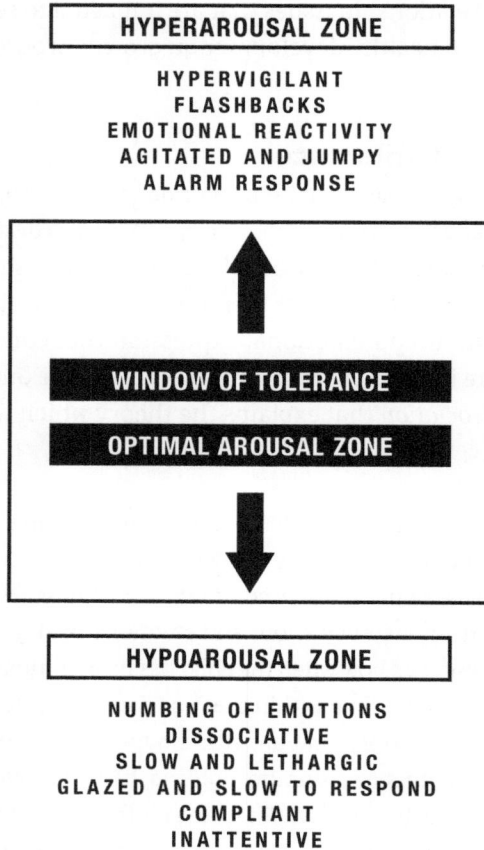

WINDOW OF TOLERANCE (FOSHA, SIEGEL AND SOLOMON, 2009)

When a child is overwhelmed, it takes them outside their Window of Tolerance. Children who are exposed to continual threat have smaller Windows of Tolerance, can become sensitive to all perceived signs of danger and can quickly move outside their windows to hypoaroused or hyperaroused behaviours to help them survive the threat. When they are outside their window, they cannot integrate their experiences due to the overwhelm and therefore they can become disintegrated memories.

## Neurodiversity

It is important to mention here that while there is a sense of what 'normal' developmental behaviour and progression are, all children are different, and a trauma-informed culture is one where we celebrate each child's individuality. This includes their individual talents and opinions and the way they view the world. Some children will have some specific neurodiversity which can be viewed as an additional challenge or as an additional gift. Neurodiversity includes different diagnoses, including dyslexia, dyspraxia, autism and many others. Research is increasing in this field, including the link with trauma, and Kalisch *et al.* (2021, p.1) assert that there is a 'high degree of overlap, co-occurrence, and shared interpersonal trauma vulnerability between children with autism and intellectual disability'.

The research also found that neurodiverse children are at heightened risk of experiencing trauma 'and are approximately two or three times more likely to encounter traumatic events of an interpersonal nature relative to their typically developing counterparts'.

This book is focused on trauma recovery and as the child, whether neurodiverse or not, is able to heal and recover from what didn't happen to them that should have happened or what did happen that should not have, the trauma symptoms should reduce.

## Normal behaviours that can be difficult for adults

Let's look at some of the primary behaviours that occur at different stages of childhood and how they may be viewed as symptoms of distress unless we are familiar with the knowledge around child development theory. With this knowledge, we can then become reassured that what might look like behaviour to worry about could in fact be entirely normal and natural and a stage that they need to progress through in order to mature in a healthy way.

### Emotional regulation and meltdowns

A child first begins to demonstrate a lack of ability to regulate their emotions from birth. They are entirely dependent on adults to co-regulate with them, and without an adult to soothe, comfort, explain, narrate and

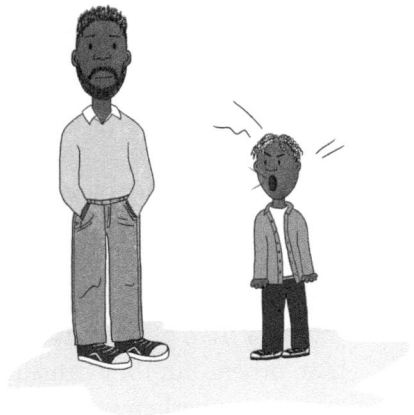

help, they can demonstrate behaviour and emotional expression that is interruptive and demonstrative. A child needs to experience continual co-regulation in the context of a few familiar and known adults whom the child has learned to trust.

If the child has had enough co-regulation, they eventually learn to regulate their own emotions without such emotional support from a familiar adult. This is emotional self-regulation. Music (2019) asserts that 'securely attached children, who generally have experienced sensitive attunement, tend automatically to develop an ability to self-regulate' (p.106). This, of course, does not mean that if they get kicked by another child or if they fall off their bike or they have to wait for what seems like an eternity for something they really want, they will be able to be 'fine'! However, a healthy child will be able to express appropriate emotion, understand what emotion it is and eventually use words to describe how they feel and then get their needs met in that moment. After many, many repetitions of co-regulation, the ability to self-regulate becomes an automatic reaction for a child because it is a well-trodden path through childhood, which leads to adults being mostly able to be socially appropriate even with feelings that can feel intense. They can excuse themselves and take a break outside, go and cry in a private space, ring a friend to process verbally or go on a run to lose some of the excess adrenaline from the conflict or challenge.

Being self-regulated doesn't mean you never have an emotional meltdown or express emotion in a demonstrative way. That could be due to the severity of the experience or due to the personality of the child. It's not abnormal until it becomes frequent and interruptive to the child's learning and ability to enjoy life.

Therefore, when a child is unable to regularly demonstrate self-regulation, we recognize that there was probably some kind of unfinished developmental process that needs to be completed. This can be completed with an adult who is able to repeatedly co-regulate with the child until they can do so on their own. A lot of teaching assistants and learning support assistants at school are functioning in that role currently. Some children are biologically less confident and natural in this area than others, just as some children are better at art or sports than others, but they can all learn to regulate with enough consistent repeated experiences that rewire their neural pathways.

The continuous and repetitive co-regulation between a parent or carer and the baby or toddler helps them lay down patterns, which naturally develop into self-regulation of their emotions and reactions. These experiences are full of oxytocin release and develop the orbitofrontal cortex. Cozolino (2006) speaks of the experience of healthy attachment relationships where it is: 'the day-to-day experience of young children as they go through cycles of regulation, dysregulation and regulation, their parents serving as external frontal lobes, helping them to navigate their emotional ups and downs of life. Repeating this experience thousands of times creates an unconscious experience of regulation' (2006, p.260). (de Thierry, 2019, p.39)

## When a child is stressed

It is normal for a child to sometimes experience stress, and that can serve as an opportunity for them to practise and strengthen their ability to explore what they may be feeling or experiencing with their attachment figure. If we recognize that it is often hard being a human of any age, then we can create space for all ages to process and try and make sense of how they feel and what went wrong or what went right but was still disappointing. We are naturally collaborative as humans and need others to remain healthy, and therefore, isolation, independence and self-obsession can cause longer-term challenges. Normal stress that seems relatively unavoidable without special treatment should not be avoided but should be approached with appropriate discussion on what is the best way to do the intimidating task. Any discussion with the child needs to be in a comfy place, often while they are doing something else that they enjoy, making sure we remain as calm as possible but giving voice to negative emotions rather than denying them or supressing them.

As adults, we can model approaching stress to the children around us by using words to explain what emotions we feel and what our bodies feel like, along with what we have planned to do to enable us to complete the task despite those feelings. We can model that they act as useful guides that we don't want to ignore, but we can use our mind to decide what to do. It is also good to explain that we have used our imagination to ponder on what would happen if things do go badly wrong, and we have also used our imagination to think about if it went well and how pleased we may feel.

As adults, when we do express emotions and the children see that, it's important not to pretend we are fine. Instead, we should use emotional language to explain what is going on so that they are not scared of what could happen but are curious and kind. We don't want them to feel responsible for us as adults, but we do want them to develop empathy for all humans who are facing challenges and big emotions.

A child's stress can be monitored, and as adults, we need to work out when we can reduce the stress and when we think the stressful experience could be of benefit to the child to learn to practise some techniques that will help them for the rest of their lives.

## Sensitive children

Some children are more sensitive than others, especially those who will become our future adult artists, musicians, dancers and creatives. They can be more sensitive to sensory and emotional experiences such as criticism or the atmosphere of a room or a messy space or noisy classroom. They may need additional support in processing some experiences, especially ones that provoke an emotional reaction. These are the children who have an emotional reaction when they hear a piece of music or are captivated by a painting or a dance that seems to take their breath away. These children can be sensitive to things that other children may rarely even notice. This element of who they are doesn't need medicating or healing; it needs adapting to. A child who is visually sensitive may need longer in an art gallery or to finish their painting in an art lesson, and may have a disproportionate reaction to not having enough time. If the teacher reports the emotional reaction of the child without the context, the parent or other staff may perceive that child to be in some way 'disordered', but when we know the context, we may feel that we have a little peep into the possible creative future they have, which will benefit us all.

If a child struggles to work in a classroom next to the toilet and is often more restless than when they are learning in other classrooms, we could assume that they have a more heightened sensitivity to smell than other children. This is why it's helpful to remember that everyone is unique and naturally has different sensitivities and interests, passions and desires, and that's what makes the world an amazing place.

Every child can be easily hurt by damaging relationships, rejection, hurtful words, nasty experiences, betrayal, insecurity, uncertainty or other such frightening experiences. However, each child will respond differently and the depth of impact will depend on several factors, including the child's primary relationships and personality. Some are much more sensitive than others and will have less resilience (i.e., ability to recover from difficult experiences), due to their character, which may be inherited or influenced by experience. For example, a child who struggles to join in group activities can also struggle to build a sense of self-confidence and this can be for a number of reasons. (de Thierry, 2017, p.14)

## Doing what they don't always want to do

It is also important to remember that many children do not want to do what they know they are expected to do, because part of the natural development of a human is the essential process of testing boundaries and seeing what is moveable and what is not. It's important for children to learn appropriate boundaries and, as Gabor Maté (1999) says:

We do not find out the boundaries of acceptable behaviour by reading a manual or even by being told. The setting of limits has to begin long before we understand why those limits must be respected. We find out by the reactions of our parents, the most important of which are non-verbal. (p.134)

It is a primary element of parenting and can sometimes be a difficult path to walk. While we want to avoid making our children feel that they have to completely conform and we want to celebrate their individuality, we also want them to take their place in society and be a helpful member of the population. We have to be mindful of the worries and reactions of each child regarding any expectations and know when the demand is too hard for them and may hurt them, and when actually they need us to push them a little to do things that may at first feel uncomfortable. Without encouragement, most of the children and adults who have achieved some kind of perceived success in musical, academic, creative, technological and inventive areas would have wanted, at some point in the process, to give up. That is a part of being human. I have almost given up many things in my 50 years of life, and I am glad I didn't, despite the pain and courage it has sometimes taken me to keep going.

Most children have days or weeks of not wanting to go to school. Many children sometimes don't want to learn or do what they are told. That is quite natural. I have certainly found it a tough element of parenting when a child says they are too unwell to go to school, but it is 7am and I can't imagine any of us feeling very well that early in the morning. I am left to try and do the best thing and guess if they really are unwell or if they have a maths test that they would like to avoid! What I do know is that I would change my mind at any point if it was clear that they were unwell when eating breakfast or on the journey to school. However, there have been many other times when they needed to chat about a test or a difficult situation they were keen to avoid at school, and at the end of the day felt relieved they had gone in.

Working out when to help the child avoid things that are difficult and when to encourage them to persevere despite the discomfort is a tough part of parenting, and we will all make mistakes. It can be helpful to talk to other parents or carers to see if something may be going on which is adding to the situational distress that the child is speaking of. Sometimes we need to do some detective work, which is worth it to help them to do things that are hard but don't put them in a space of deep distress.

'I assumed that I didn't need to know much anyway so I couldn't see the point of learning what seemed to be stupid stuff. Now I regret not knowing more about the things other kids seemed to learn at school. But I couldn't concentrate because I was too terrified of what was happening at home. So, I just got through. No one told me I was clever and helped me understand why learning this stuff could be helpful one day!' *Pete, now aged 21*

## A child's relationships

Wouldn't it be so simple if a child made a group of friends and they were able to stay with the same group all the way through their childhood? Sadly, this does not happen as much as television shows make it appear. Children move homes and schools, children change their interests or hobbies, and situations change, which means that relationships change.

It is not always easy to watch children navigate their way through friendship challenges, and it can also remind many of us of the negative experiences we had to go through. It is normal, however, for children to sometimes feel as if they don't have friends or for them to feel they are no longer a valued part of a friendship group that was an essential part of their life. It's up to us as the adults to help them express the emotions of loss, grief and sadness about the changes. We can also help them explore who they do feel some kind of connection with and help them with ideas of how to play or spend time with some other children who seem to be friends with them. Again, once the child heads towards puberty, we need to take a step back and let them lead the navigation, with our role being to support them emotionally and remain a solid, consistent, loving figure in their life.

Children need help with their relationships and rarely can they navigate all 18 or so years without support from their adults. Let's normalize this and recognize that popular comedies like *Friends* have caused a great deal of misrepresentation of the reality of the complexity of relationships.

## The development of identity

There are many strong views and psychological theories on how personality is formed through childhood. Ultimately, a child is influenced by their experiences and emotional reactions to those, their attachment relationships, other adults in their life, such as teachers or activity group leaders, and their friends. These people all influence who the child thinks they are and how they feel they are perceived by society. Waters (2016) asserts that 'a person's identity is shaped by human experiences and interpersonal interactions, in which new experiences are continually being assimilated, resulting in solidifying, modifying, or disrupting earlier patterns of beliefs, affect and behaviour' (p.38).

Sadly, we can see that now screens and social media have a greater influence on the child if they have access to them without strong restrictions. The influence of strangers on social media includes many adults who are purposefully aiming to shape children's identity and cause insecurity and distress. This is leading to a fast-rising population of children who are worrying about things that years ago weren't in the minds or conversations of children until they were past puberty and had greater capacity to understand and comprehend the world.

It is normal for a child to:

- look into a mirror and feel insecure about some aspect of themselves
- worry that they aren't normal
- want to look like someone more popular or clever
- express sadness that they aren't like someone else
- want to be someone else, or prettier or more handsome.

All of these normal feelings don't have to become influential in their life and can become passing moments when they have an adult who has a strong attachment relationship with them and is able to reassure them and tell stories of when they were young or of things they wanted to change that they are now glad they instead grew to like.

## Conclusion

As adults, we need to know when to worry about the child or when they are just going through a normal phase of development. We need to learn from people who have dedicated their lives to studying and researching humans and have discovered themes and patterns in thousands of children across many decades. It can be really tough to be the primary support of a child unless we also have support from others who have a track record of enabling many children to develop into confident adults.

## Questions to reflect on
### For parents/carers/therapeutic mentors

- What behaviours have you worried about, and do you think they may be normal for the age of the child?
- What behaviours did you show as a child that were probably normal?
- Have you seen children panicking about 'having anxiety issues' or 'anger management issues' when they are expressing fear or

anger in a normal way? What could we do as adults to reassure them?

- Which 'normal' behaviour for children is one that you struggle with the most when a child is like that?
- What behaviour is normal for you when you are stressed? What about children? When should we be concerned about their behaviour?
- Are you aware of any sensitive children? How do they react when they feel unsafe or scared? What do you think they may need?
- How does identity form over the years? What developments are quite normal? What does child development theory suggest is the age at which children can make decisions that they have to live with for the rest of their lives?

## For therapists

- What subtle signals do you note when 'normal behaviour' now shows distress?
- What child development theorist do you refer back to as a way to reflect on behaviour and distress?
- Have you reflected on or wrestled with the current culture that seems to be communicating that children need a diagnosis to validate behaviour that can be normal? What do you think?
- What do you say to the adults who are concerned about the normal behaviour being a sign of a diagnosis needed?

# CHAPTER 3

# Relationships That Can Facilitate Healing

## Feeling connected and feeling alive

As humans, we need connection with others to stay alive. Trauma is an experience that confuses, distorts and injures our connection with others, and the impact is that the traumatized person often feels less alive and instead scared and numb. One of the main impacts of trauma is disconnection with others and disconnection with ourselves. Therefore, the primary route to healing must be built on the foundation of relationships that are therapeutic and nurturing to help the person begin to come back to life again.

López-Zerón and Blow (2015) researched the impact of relationships for a traumatized person and found that 'close relationships can maintain or exacerbate problems, but they can also be a powerful source of healing'. When a child feels disconnected from others, it often causes a disconnection internally, which further escalates trauma symptoms as the child struggles to push through survival while feeling alone and rejected. This is called dissociation and can escalate the more they feel pressured to carry on as if they are 'normal'. Dissociation and how to facilitate recovery from that will be explored briefly in Section 3 and is discussed more thoroughly in the book *The Simple Guide to Complex Trauma and Dissociation*.

There are vastly different experiences of trauma and different reactions and symptoms, but one thing they all have in common is the need for positive, emotionally intelligent attachment relationships that can be a 'safe place' for the child to begin to recover.

## The role of a primary attachment figure

To understand how healing and restoration can be facilitated for a traumatized person, it is vital to understand the theories around attachment. Attachment theory focuses on the need for proximity to a sensitive caregiver in childhood who provides a sense of security and a safe base from which to explore the world. Gabor Maté (1999) says that 'being wanted and enjoyed is the greatest gift the child can receive. It is the basis of self-acceptance' (p.154). One of my other books, *The Simple Guide to Attachment Difficulties* (2019), explores at greater length the role of the attachment figure and how relational trauma can be healed through relational connection, but because it is so central to all trauma recovery work, here is a brief overview.

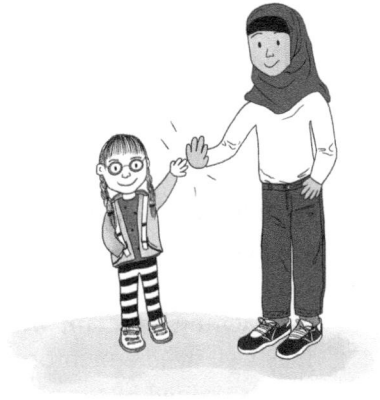

> Attachment is a word that is used to describe the ability to enable a child to feel emotionally and physically safe through their relationship with their 'main adult(s)' who cares for them. Attachment theory was first developed by a psychologist called John Bowlby (1988), who was fascinated by the early relationship between babies and their mother and how much that affected them as they grew up. The concept has developed from being solely about a mother and her baby to cover the whole experience of a child's ability to feel intrinsically emotionally safe with their primary carer(s). (de Thierry, 2019, p.13)

Many children experience difficulties in forming that vital attachment relationship with a primary caregiver due to the trauma experience that is impacting them all. For example, a child may be living in a chaotic home, with domestic abuse or violence; they may be living in desperation, with poverty and homelessness; their primary attachment figure may have unprocessed childhood trauma; the adult may be struggling with physical or mental illness or may have other traumatic experiences that mean they are in survival mode and find it hard to be emotionally available enough to build a relationship where the child can feel safe. There is no blame or shame towards that parent, and it is usually not too late to try and rebuild the relationship if the child is pre-puberty. After puberty, it can be more difficult to rebuild a broken or negative attachment relationship, but it can still be possible.

## The adult team around the child

Ideally, for a child to recover from trauma, they need several adults to help them. They need a primary attachment figure and then a teacher or teaching assistant with whom they can feel safe at school. They may well need a mentor or a therapeutic helper or a psychotherapist who is trained in a trauma recovery model such as my TRFM® to help them process the trauma. Appropriate communication between the adults is essential, so that together they can monitor any changes to the child's behaviour or any new stressors that arise. As they work together as a team, focusing on building relationships where the child feels safe, known and cared for, the child can slowly begin to untangle their insides, which can feel like tangled ball of rubbish that they are holding on to because it is all they have ever known.

Some primary caregivers of the child feel an urgency to know all that happens in therapy and preferably be present for the sessions. I would assert that sometimes the child needs the space to explore and process different experiences in a messy way with someone who isn't going to be a long-term relationship, so that they can then bring the more processed story or experience or thought to the primary caregiver. It's not so much that the primary caregiver is able to say that they can 'cope' and 'would rather know all the mess'; it's more about the child and their need to have a little sense of control when they have been powerlessness for so long. Most of us would want some of our worst moments to be airbrushed before those around us knew of them and could offer support. Therapy can offer the child that experience so that there is strong and positive communication with the primary caregiver and attachment figure, but there is also a sense of privacy and space to explore mess with no long-term repercussions. This is especially important in the older years as the child progresses towards adolescence,

*The more positive relationships the child has, the easier it will be for*

*them to recover.* Let's explore how these relationships can facilitate elements of trauma recovery.

## Therapists and therapeutic professionals working together

It is important to note that while the therapeutic mentor can facilitate the building of relationships, psychoeducation, safety and stability work that is the foundation for trauma recovery, the processing of trauma needs to be facilitated by a professional who is trained as a clinician. A psychologist or psychotherapist needs to lead the trauma processing, which cannot be done safely until the foundations of safety and stability are built. The ideal team around the child is like the team that would be present if they needed a medical operation in a hospital. They need the supportive adult who attends the hospital with them and co-regulates, comforts, soothes and reassures them. They need the team of nurses to administer medication and offer suggestions for how to reduce the risk of infection, and they need the surgeons who do the operation. The therapist is the equivalent of the surgeon and is needed alongside the therapeutic professionals who nurse and care for the child, with the parent or carer as the adult who offers all-round care, following through the treatment plan written by the nurse and surgeon.

## Emotional connection

Children need to feel seen, heard and valued by the adults who are responsible for caring for them. Children experience the adults around them even before birth though the sounds and feeling within the womb, and the first five years are foundational for healthy development of their understanding of what to expect in the world from adults. If the adult is stressed, overwhelmed, not well or has not had experiences of emotional connection themselves, it can be difficult for them to offer emotional connection. The child views the need for emotional connection as life-giving and the fear of it being withdrawn as a threat to life. Emotional connection with a child is developed through repeated experiences of the adult being warm, nurturing, playful and kind and when the adult is able to attune to the needs of the child and respond to what they think may be going on when there aren't many words to bring clarity.

**The Six C's of Co-regulating with a child**

Care

Connect

Co-regulate

Calm

Comfort

Consider

THE SIX C'S OF CO-REGULATING WITH A CHILD © BETSY DE THIERRY 2023 (DE THIERRY, 2023)

**TRFM® TOOL 3**: The Six C's of Co-Regulating with a Child

Children and young people who have experienced trauma often have extreme emotional reactions that can lead to challenging behaviour. How do they begin to regulate these emotions?

These C's are in sequential order. In other words, the child needs to experience the first C before they can feel the next one.

**Care:** The child needs to sense that you like them, care for them and want the best for them. Without that as a starting point, it's almost impossible for them to want to move to connecting with you at all. They will often assume that they are not worthy of being liked by you or that you find them annoying.

**Connect:** Once they feel that you genuinely care for them, then they will be able to slowly begin to emotionally connect with you. They will begin to like being with you and feel a warm sense of acceptance.

**Co-regulate:** From that place, they will be more able to let you co-regulate them, which means that you can use your voice to 'wonder out loud' what may be going on when they feel upset or dysregulated, and you can help them with emotional language that expresses how they feel in a less destructive way than they may be used to!

**Calm:** Only when they have had repeated experiences over a long time of the first three C's will they be able to experience what calm feels like, without it feeling uncomfortable.

**Comfort:** From a place of feeling relatively calm, they can then be introduced to sensory experiences that bring a sense of comfort.

**Consider:** It's only when the other C's have been repeated and experienced that the child is usually ready and able to consider what happened and why, and even be able to offer some reconciliation or restoration.

If we rush children through this, it can become an unpleasant and fake experience of an adult 'making them do something', which can cause them to subconsciously view adults as not genuine and therefore see themselves as not worthy of care. The six C's have to be experienced over time, with adults who are prepared to be as consistent as possible and offer a genuine apology when it doesn't go as well as they had hoped.

My six C's are in sequential order and help us remember that if we first show that we care through our facial reactions, body language, tone of voice and words, it enables us to connect with them. From this connection, we are able to co-regulate, calm, comfort and then gently help them consider what has been going on and how they may be feeling.

When the adult is able to be repeatedly emotionally available for the child, the consequence is that the child doesn't need to use subconscious or conscious coping mechanisms to cope with their daily new experiences and emotions, but are able instead to relax back into the safety and trust of their parent. When there has been an interruption to the positive emotional connection in the relationship, this can be repaired in the same way that a lot of other relational restoration occurs – through repetitive positive relational experiences, alongside the ability to create space to reflect on things that haven't gone so well.

## Empathy is a must for emotional connection

Empathy is another way to begin to offer emotional connection and it can begin when the child is not present. Brené Brown (2021) says:

> We need to dispel the myth that empathy is 'walking in someone else's shoes.' Rather than walking in your shoes, I need to learn how to listen to the story you tell about what it's like in your shoes and believe you even when it doesn't match my experiences. (p.123)

This takes courage and emotional capacity because to reflect on what the child experiences in their life, we have to feel it enough ourselves to grasp what could be their worst fear or their greatest delight; to reflect on what it would feel like for them to have their nightmares come true or to have their dreams come true. This is the hard work of taking the time to get to know the child and be able to care for them and help them navigate through triggering experiences. Empathy is not sympathy, where we look on and feel sorry for the person but avoid taking the time and emotional energy to reflect on their experience. It takes courage and maturity to put our own experiences and filter away so we can wonder what it may be like to be them. This can happen when we listen to them enough to be able to imagine what they may feel like and what may be the things that terrify them.

It takes us time and courage to reflect on the darkness that they have endured, but there is no other way of forming a bridge into their lives to be able to reach them with our care and nurture.

To be able to emotionally connect with a child, we first must take time to consider who they are. We can reflect on different questions such as:

- What do they love and what do they hate?
- What was the worst thing that happened to them and how might they have felt at the time and then felt afterwards?
- What would be their greatest delight? How would they express it?
- What would be the best day or the worst day for them?
- What are they scared about?
- What do they especially want their adults around them to know about them?

As we begin to wonder about how they survived and where there may be shame or fear of rejection or fear of failure or terror of things like their traumatic experience happening again, we can begin to tread more carefully and naturally feel more sensitivity about the things that they feel sensitive about.

## Attunement is a central skill

Attunement is the process of emotionally connecting to the other person by noticing their facial reaction, tone of voice and body posture while listening to them. It is a vital element for all relationships to have a sense of flow and ease rather than feeling uncomfortable and awkward.

> Attunement is a way of tuning into the other person and how they are feeling and is an important skill to use when relating to babies, children and others. It's the ability to notice how the person or people around us are feeling or responding and then reacting accordingly. A well attuned person notices the unspoken emotional state of the other person and adapts their emotions, moods, body language, tone of voice and general responses to be able to communicate with them in a way that enables emotional connection. (de Thierry, 2019, p.26)

When a child feels the comfortable rhythm of a relationship with an adult where the pace, interactions, environment and activities are either fun and enjoyable or helpful and thought provoking or both, the child develops stronger relationship muscles, which then positively impact all other relationships. Without relationship practice from adults, the child will never learn how to build emotional connections which help them feel known, valued and alive. As humans, it is, of course, impossible to be perfect in many areas of relationship, including being emotionally attuned all the time. In fact, if we try too hard, we may become unpleasant to be around due to our hidden stress and desperation to be perfect! Music (2019) helps all primary caregivers with the encouraging words that:

> mother-infant interactions are rarely smooth. Tronick (2007) suggested that good mutual attunement occurs only about 30% of the time in the

best mother-infant relationship! It is the repair of misattunements that leads to resilience, when ruptures are not too catastrophic and repairs are good and quick enough. (p.36)

The repair of ruptures and misattunement moments can build stronger relationships when the adult is speedy enough to notice and seek out a repair in an authentic, genuine, kind and honest way.

## Attuning to the adult

A child is desperate to trust the adults around them, but they are also terrified of being hurt or scared more than they already have been. They are therefore usually sensitive or hypervigilant to the non-verbal communication of adults, which is found in facial expressions, tone of voice, eye movements, emotional expression in the voice or bodily movements, and it is here that they decide if the adult is 'safe' or not. Our nervous system is an area within all relationships that we cannot pretend about easily. A traumatized child or an attuned child will be able to pick up the state of an adult's nervous system quickly and will react to what they feel. It may not be visible to others looking on at a distance and could be hidden under a smile or jokes or playful activities, but children quickly pick up on the mood or vibe of an adult. If the adult feels anxious and is agitated or unsettled, the child will pick up on that more than anything said. If the adult tries to reassure the child that they are relaxed, but the hypervigilant child can tell that they are not, then the child is likely to say that they just don't want to be in the company of that adult. They will be unlikely to use words expressing concern or discomfort about the adult's nervous system, but they will be reticent to engage in authentic conversation or activities if they sense this invisible but powerful dysregulation in the adult. Ultimately, fear, distress, anxiety, sadness can all be transferred through emotional contagion to the child because children are learning about the world and are curious about other people in order to understand them better.

When adults are struggling with fear or anxiety, it is usually better for them to say to the child something like 'I'm just feeling a little anxious this morning, but I will try and do my breathing exercises and have a hot drink and then I hope I will be fine. You don't have to worry, though...' This enables the child to feel that they have permission to not like the feeling they could pick up on and that they also don't have to take responsibility for the adult. Otherwise, anxious adults often have anxious children despite the best intentions.

## Validation

Validation is another tool in our toolbox. When a child expresses an opinion, names an emotion, explains something or wants to show their adult something, it is an opportunity to validate them. Validation is the feeling of being noticed, understood and connected. Sometimes, as adults, we need to share how tough an experience was so that some-one can validate our experience with a story that describes how awful they found a similar experience. We can seek out validation and so can children.

When people experience the opposite of validation, it drives them away from connection with that person as they feel misunderstood, disconnected and invalidated. For example, when people say things like this it can cause huge pain and distress:

I had it worse when I was young.

You are just too sensitive and need to grow up.

Why can't you be like (your sister/brother/a friend)?

Why can't you just move on as it was ages ago that bad thing happened?

You are lying about what happened – it wasn't like that/or that bad.

Validation is about acknowledging that the emotion or sensation is a felt experience – even if it doesn't make much sense. When a person feels validated, they are then able to reflect and sometimes change their mind about what they are feeling, but if they are fighting to have the warm and relieving feeling of being seen and validated, then they could remain stubborn and assert their rights rather than gently lean in to acknowledge their feelings. It's not about logic and being 'right', but about being heard and seen and listened to. (de Thierry, 2023, p.97)

61

As memories of the trauma become stories that need to be put into words, they seem to become more real and no longer like a dream. This can feel like a shock. Often, survivors of trauma are told they exaggerate or are liars, and so when someone shows validation and empathy and even expresses their own pain over what has happened to the child, it can begin to break the silence of the lie that maybe it was their fault and maybe they exaggerated. Validation is the ability to communicate through words, tone of voice and body language that you believe the child is communicating to the best of their ability what they remember happened and how it made them feel. People who have survived trauma need repeated validation in order to know that they are believed and that it is wrong that they had to suffer.

It is important to remember to validate strongly and repeatedly the feelings that need to be expressed about what happened. At the same time, we also need to carefully balance this with the need for the child to want to move forward towards growth and recovery. Validating trauma symptoms continually can cause them to become 'stuck in self-defeating behaviour patterns that are no longer adaptive' (Silberg, 2012, p.55).

> 'I didn't know that other children didn't worry about answering questions about what was happening at home. I could never say what was going on because I don't know what would have happened if I did. I just felt stuck so would lie and avoid adults talking to me.'
> Amy, aged 12

## Slowing down to build positive relationships

The world seems to be in such a rush and people seem to be constantly busy and aiming to achieve more things in their days. This is leading to many people feeling surrounded by people but not feeling known, seen or heard, and not knowing how to find the space to experience those things. Children are showing their distress at the pace of things and are reacting to additional pressure in different ways, but they rarely have words to describe what they feel.

Ultimately, children of all ages flourish when they can enjoy simple things that require the adults to slow down to enjoy them with them. This can be seen as the fuel of a positive healing relationship.

Rather than constantly ticking off the next lists of attainments that the child needs to complete, it works better when there is a slowing down and the child can begin to learn how to do simple things at a pace that feels calm and comforting. Children who have experienced stress, violence, terror, war, assault, chaos and other terrifying and unrelenting experiences may find this really hard at first. It can feel unfamiliar to be in a calm, gentle and fun environment. Humans are usually drawn to that which feels familiar, even if it is uncomfortable or painful, and unfamiliar environments can feel scary and so can often be something to try and avoid. The slower pace can become a new familiar once it is a repeated, positive experience and has the power to gradually change the child's internal heightened rhythm of chaos.

As psychotherapists working with children, we intentionally walk a little slower, watch the child notice things and notice them too. We allow the child to quietly and slowly explore the room, as they look for signs of safety or danger. As we slow down to notice what they notice, and as we notice our own nervous system and are mindful of our breath, we can facilitate the child to do so too. We often have a long treatment plan to fulfil, with aims and objectives, and we share a desperation for the child to experience stability, regulation and restoration, and this fuels the appointment, but it's mostly in the slow, steady pace that healing begins to unfold.

Finding activities to do which both the supporting adult or parent and the child enjoy is also critical as it is time spent with positive emotional contagion and calm or excited nervous system reactions. Research has shown the value of playing with children and how that enables connection and learning in a way that is positive and healing. 'Play activities can be used both as an emotional state change strategy and as occasions for experimentation with positive effects, regulation, and connection' (D'Elia, Carpinelli & Savarese, 2022). These moments of shared play build relationships and positive memories and are worth using emotional energy to invest in regularly.

When we as the adult can offer this kind of relationship, we are offering hope for recovery.

The TRFM® emotional connection model to help you quickly remember the main elements of connecting:

## CURIOUS MODEL

**C** Curious and kind.

**U** Unrushed and available.

**R** Regulated nervous system.

**I** Interested in their interests.

**O** Open face and tone of voice.

**U** Unconditional warmth and belief in them.

**S** Shame reducing.

CURIOUS MODEL © BETSY DE THIERRY 2025

**TRFM® TOOL 4: Curious Model**

## How authentic can I be?

As an adult, emotional connection with others needs to be something that has been developed in the context of other relationships. Children need us to have grown confident in who we are and how to be ourselves around others. Being authentic is essential because children cannot feel connected to an adult who seems to be acting out a role; they will notice if the adult is trying too hard or is not really pleased to be there. This makes them feel disconnected. A child who is traumatized is hypersensitive to the adults around them and knows instinctively who they feel safe with. Research confirms that 'maltreated children exhibit enhanced sensitivity to negative facial expressions, including a biased tendency to classify emotions as negative when categorizing emotional facial expressions' (Masten *et al.*, 2008). When an adult displays facial reactions that they perceive as neutral, it is important to recognize that they can be seen as negative by children who have experienced trauma. An adult supporter should not cross appropriate boundaries around the role of supporting the child, and therefore should not share their struggles or worries with them, because the child needs to believe that the adult has the emotional resilience or strength to support them. If the child senses that their adult is not coping and needs support, they may express anger towards them because they need a strong and reliable person on whom they feel they can off-load some of the weight they are carrying, and who won't get crushed by what they share.

## What if the primary adult is unpredictable?

Sometimes, the main parent or carer of the child who has experienced trauma is also traumatized and therefore may be struggling with their own symptoms. When the primary adult is navigating their own way through to trauma recovery, they may be experienced by the child as unpredictable because the child needs an emotionally available, calm adult. It is important that the child has access to another consistent, long-term, predictable adult so that any negative experiences they have of the unpredictable adult can be explored and processed. Predictable adult supporters are needed to build a stable and emotionally safe foundation for the child to heal and recover from trauma, and so, for many families, we need to pioneer ways to help them while reducing the shame of needing support and being intentional about building safe and consistent communities.

## Controlling adults

It is important to note that because the nature of supporting a child through to trauma recovery is volatile and chaotic and exhausting, the adult may begin to want to control the child, their other relationships, their activities, their food and drink, their therapeutic support and anything else where the adult thinks their relationship could be threatened. Some parents may be trying to provide the opposite of their childhood experience of neglect and do not realize that the level of control is causing similar trauma impact. Control is a deeply damaging experience for the child who becomes further powerless, dehumanized and disconnected.

Victims often describe coercive control as not being 'allowed', or having to ask permission, to do everyday things; and being in constant fear of not meeting the abuser's expectations or complying with their demands. The term 'walking on eggshells' is often used. (McLeod & Flood, 2018)

The child needs to be able to be heard, to see the adult change their mind after listening carefully, and needs to understand that other adults offering support generally doesn't decrease the vital role of the adult but instead offers additional support. If a child feels that they are 'owned' by their primary caregiver or that they must fulfil a need within them, they will not be able to begin to recover from trauma but instead may pretend to comply while internally disconnecting and breeding a sense of hatred. They would rarely be able to offer you any hint that they may be feeling that if you asked, because control over children becomes the primary trauma they experience as they deeply desire to be able to make their own decisions and have their opinion and hunches validated. Coercive control can lead to mind control, which renders the child unable to function independently unless they are doing what their adult wants, due to feeling terrified and helpless. They also feel disconnected to others and confused about their place in the world. As a vital element of caring for them, children need to be empowered to reflect, offer their views and be heard.

## Conclusion

Relationships are the thread that is found within every aspect of trauma recovery. Becoming more skilled at emotional connection through attunement, empathy, compassion, listening skills, being emotionally available, being calm despite the chaos and going at a gentle pace with a nervous system that is as regulated as possible is the primary foundation that recovery can be built on.

## Questions to reflect on
### For parents/carers/therapeutic mentors

- Who is the child's primary attachment figure?

- What could be done to strengthen that relationship?
- What is currently the biggest challenge to that becoming a healing relationship?
- What other relationships does this child have that are positive? How can they remain a priority for the family?
- What other professionals are involved in the child's life?
- Which ones are helpful towards the goal of trauma recovery?
- Which ones are not helpful and what could you do to resource them, train them, remove them?
- What do you think your child's understanding of relationships is at the moment?
- How can you monitor that changing for the better so that the foundation is prepared for healing?

## For therapists

- How are you finding working with the team around the family? Is there good communication and could you strengthen the sense of trust, empathy and kindness within the team?
- How are you managing the impact of empathy in your role as you stand in the shoes of so many traumatic experiences? How are you discharging those feelings so that they don't negatively impact you?

CHAPTER 4

# Environments That Facilitate Healing

While relationships are the key foundation for all trauma recovery, a physically and emotionally safe, predictable environment is also vital for the journey. When children spend time in environments where there seems to be no order, no sense of predictability or calm and no clear boundaries to keep them safe, they can feel further powerless and overwhelmed. While there are some environments that cannot be altered to serve the needs of traumatized children who are seeking to recover from the symptoms that now debilitate them, we know that other environments can be changed when there is understanding. This area is another vital step to enable the trauma recovery journey to be embarked on. 'A safe, predictable environment helps traumatized children to relax defences, learn from their experiences, and trust that their needs will be met' (Waters, 2016, p.135).

## Physically safe

An environment that is physically safe enables the child to trust that they won't be physically harmed by being there. It is a place where the adults have reflected on risk and made decisions that enable children to play and enjoy the space because the risks have been minimized. For example, an adult may reflect about the elements of a garden, such as a fence or gate that stops the toddler running onto the road. It could be that adults have made sure that things like wires and other trip hazards have been secured to the wall, so children won't fall over. A physically safe environment is a trauma-informed space because empathy has been used to reflect on what harm could be caused and what could stop that risk. Thought has gone into how the space could be used to facilitate play and calm so that it supports a child beginning to move out of fear and defence into a calm and connected state. Physically safe environments are places and spaces where there is reduced potential for physical harm, threat or violence.

## Classrooms

While most classrooms cannot remain consistently calm, the child who has experienced trauma is usually on high alert for any sign of danger that could cause them to feel terror, powerlessness and overwhelm, and so they remain hypervigilant and ready to respond to the threat that may be awaiting them. If a child is twitchy, agitated or looks around them, if they are unsettled when the door opens or a window closes, if they look up quickly if someone coughs or moves quickly or loudly, then we recognize that they may have experienced terror in previous situations that wounded them and taught them to remain consistently alert for danger. This is called hypervigilance and is a trauma symptom, although some children who experience this are not traumatized but just more sensitive to sensory experiences.

Levine (1997) explains that humans use hypervigilance to channel some of the excess energy we have to defend ourselves against a threat, which turns into 'energy into the muscles of the head, neck, and eyes in an obsessive search for danger'. He explains what we see all the time in the lives of those who are stuck in a state of terror: that 'in the hypervigilant state, all change, including changes in our own internal states, is perceived as a threat' (p.156). If a child is finding that they are stuck in a state of hypervigilance all the time due to the unrelenting chaos of many students fighting and being distressed, then they may begin to show signs of distress.

## Hospitals and doctors' surgeries

Obviously, if a child has to have medical treatment or even visit a relative in a place such as a hospital, they can feel less than safe due to the sounds of patients in pain or crying alongside the sight of many unwell patients and professionals running around. The way to help a child navigate through those justified feelings of fear is to explain what the helpers are doing and how clever they are and how they are there to help recovery. When a child can take some comfort and sensory reminders of safety into hospital, this can help not only emotionally but also physically because we recognize that physical healing is easier when the child is more relaxed and less terrified. It can be difficult to explain to a child when they hear someone scream in pain when giving birth, that it is a positive sound of them being helped, because obviously the sound is distressing. But the child needs that reassurance and explanation; for example, when a wound needs cleaning, although it can hurt more, in the long term this allows it to heal.

For younger children, therapeutic story books about visiting hospitals can be very helpful in normalizing the strange environment. For older children, it can be beneficial for them to hear stories of other children and what they have been through and how helpful the medical intervention was for them.

Please see Chapter 21 on medical trauma for further exploration.

## Feeling sensorily safe

Neuroscientists have shown that our brain develops in childhood from the bottom to the top, and the lower brain is the part that processes sensory information – all the sights, sounds, smells and physical sensations that we may experience. The brain continues to process information in that sequential pattern and so we need to make sure that the senses feel that the environment is safe and suitable for them. This is why if you are feeling stressed and you enter a beautiful place, you may notice that you feel physically relaxed, and that will change your breathing, heart rate and how you perceive your life in that moment. As adults, we can move from a stressed state to a comfortable state quickly if the environment is changed and we experience a sense of relief. I personally find myself tidying cupboards when I am extremely stressed as I find that moving objects from chaos to order and feeling pleasure in the outcome is comforting and far easier than the work I do trying to help chaotic and traumatized families find some calm and predictability! My work team know why my head is deep in a cupboard!

If distressing noises are unavoidable, such as in spaces with younger children who may cry or have dysregulated emotional reactions that are unavoidable and unpredictable, the child can feel safe if the response from the adult to those sudden noises and movements is one of kind, confident, warm and reassuring nurture. The sound of a confident and nurturing voice instructing a class of children can help bring a sense of order and can be fascinating for a traumatized child who can eventually begin to build a sense of trust with that adult offering such nurturing care. Some children may benefit from ear defenders to help the shock of loud noises be less invasive, but many won't need them.

If distressing smells are a part of your setting, then it is important to recognize that this may have a significant impact on the behaviour or ability of the child to engage in anything positive. They will probably not be able to use their voice to explain why they feel discomfort as they may not know why, but it is vital that we recognize any toilet smells, nappy bin smells, strong food smells or other off-putting smells and plan a way to decrease the impact by opening windows and using different positive smells and methods to stop bad smells travelling through corridors.

The use of soft cushions with clean and intentional pleasant sensory experiences, blankets to stroke or snuggle in, chairs that are the right size and feel comfy and safe, pictures that feel age-appropriate and calming and are not old, worn and dusty can all help to create spaces where children feel welcomed and cared for. Broken, old toys and books that have pages missing communicate that the space is struggling to fund the support, and children can internalize thoughts that cause them to not want to add to the adult's stress. This can lead them to not feel able to explore their trauma for fear of adding further distress to a tired and exhausted-looking setting. A newly painted wall, a few clean and fresh pictures, and welcome messages along with some books and toys that are full of life can send messages that the child is welcome, and the setting is prepared to help them.

## The neuroscience around sensory information

Sensory receptors capture external stimuli from the environment (through tactile, visual, gustatory, olfactory and auditory receptors) or internal stimuli originated in our own body (via tactile, vestibular or proprioceptive receptors). These receptors transform the captured stimulus into sensory information that is sent to the brain to be processed, resulting in a determined motor and behavioural response. Sensory integration is essentially 'the neurological process that organizes sensation from one's own body and from the environment and makes it possible to use the body effectively with the environment' (Ayres, 1989).

Building on the understanding of neuroscience around the impact of trauma is Bruce Perry's neurosequential diagram of the four areas of the brain (Perry, 2014). This shows how the brainstem is at the bottom of the brain where the automatic fight, flight freeze, flop, fawn reaction is located, alongside sensory processing. Information about safety is experienced and automatically interpreted as dangerous or safe by this bottom area of the brain, which doesn't have the benefit of the higher areas of the brain that can process information and facts. The brainstem is the area of the brain where sensory information is received and acted upon instinctively. The diencephalon is the next area of the brain which enables the child to regulate usually with help from an adult. The next area of the brain is the limbic brain which enables the child to relate to other people and know how they feel about the experiences and listen and speak about what took place. Eventually, the cortex is able to process the experience and reason, so they can see that maybe they overreacted due to their brainstem getting muddled about the experience.

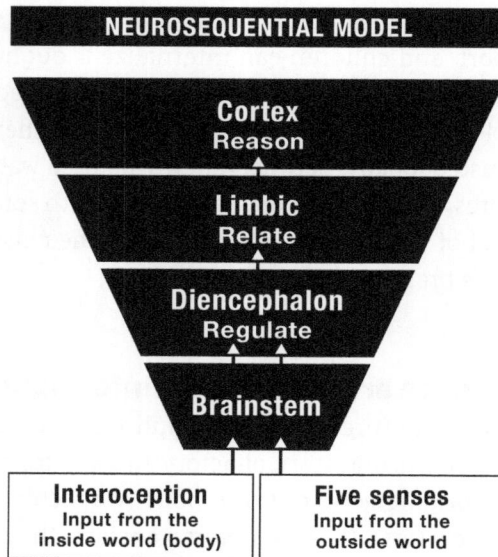

NEUROSEQUENTIAL MODEL

Cortex
Reason

Limbic
Relate

Diencephalon
Regulate

Brainstem

Interoception
Input from the
inside world (body)

Five senses
Input from the
outside world

(PERRY, 2021, P.142)

When we recognize that we each need to have access to our cortex to be able to be reasonable and rational, we can see why so many behaviours seem to shock the child who is displaying them alongside the adults around them. They often have an instinctive emotional reaction before their thinking brain has time to compute what they are doing. The brainstem holds memories of past sensory experiences and reacts from those memories, but it can't effectively match that sensory input with the current input and draw accurate conclusions. Some of us find that we match the sound of sirens with the feeling of disaster or death rather than a quick and exciting birth of a baby. We can match the sound of a slammed door with an upcoming fight rather than a surprise from a friend with boxes of birthday doughnuts or friends who slammed a door by a mistake. 'It is important to realize that children's behaviour never comes out of nowhere' (Silberg, 2012, p.138).

## An example of a sensory trigger and what could help in a classroom

A child who has been in a car accident and was taken to hospital while in pain and terror may well have an automatic brainstem reaction to the sound of the ambulance going past his school. He doesn't want to have that reaction, and his injuries weren't as bad as they may have been, and he had an enjoyable one-night stay in hospital where he ate ice cream and was given gifts for his bravery. His brainstem, however, has interpreted the ambulance as 'danger', and he wasn't able to update the information fast enough, so as the sound occurred near his classroom, he reacted as if he was dying in pain and fear.

If, however, he could have had a practised safety plan to quickly find calm in a pre-planned way, he may have found that he could use that plan instead of his dramatic explosion of dysregulated emotion due to terror. He could run to the special cushion in his classroom and find comfort from an adult, where he could then *regulate* his emotions, which is done in the diencephalon area of the brain. Once he was regulated, he could *relate* to that adult, which happens from the limbic area of the brain, and this would lead him to be able to ask what happened. In that moment, the adult could reassure him that he was safe, and that would calm his brain down enough to be able reflect and move through to *relate* and to *reason*, which is the cortex area of the brain. Here he could reflect on the sound of the ambulance and how he doesn't even mind it, and so the adult could help him draw a picture of the ambulance and tell his story to her. This will enable the unconscious experience to be made conscious, which decreases his future automatic reactions to the sound. Without a plan created in advance for him to able to run to a place that he knows is safe, such as the special cushion, he may instead escalate further in his distressed behaviour, which would cause further disruption for other children.

Children feel more empowered when they understand why their brain is reacting in ways that can sometimes embarrass them. They love to learn the neuroscience language and explain to others why humans can come to faulty conclusions due to being stuck in the primitive, automatic reaction of terror in the brainstem.

## Shame in schools

Children who have experienced developmental or complex trauma usually have a deep sense of shame because they assume on a sub-conscious and sometimes conscious level that there must be something wrong with them for these awful experiences to happen to them. Chapter 10 explores shame in more depth, but it is important to know that some educational environments are not experienced as safe due to many systems within the school that can cause further shame to children who are experiencing trauma or trying to move on from their experiences. We recognize that 'every educational opportunity offers the possibility of failure' and that 'children with core shame often struggle to participate in class, interact with peers, and feel like a part of the group' (Cozolino, 2006, p.124).

If a child is having challenges with their attachment relationships or if they are currently trying to survive trauma that cannot be spoken of yet, they can experience further terror in school. While there are many possible examples of shame-based strategies, here are some examples that can cause harm to traumatized children:

- Celebrating 100% attendance. We know that sometimes medical treatment and trauma can stop that being possible. We know that sometimes the child may be saying they feel sick because they know their bruises may be spotted from physical abuse and they can't tell someone because they are terrified. They may be terrified about failing a test and know they could be hit when the adult finds out the result. They may be caring for their parent or sibling at home. There are so many life experiences that mean we should celebrate when children get to school, at whatever time.

- Speaking about a child who is acting younger by saying 'act your age'. We know that regressive behaviour is usually due to stress or distress. It can be a significant sign of trauma or anxiety. A child naturally wants to be accepted by their peers and so will be able to 'act their age' whenever they can.
- Celebrating good behaviour and shaming those who haven't concentrated on or finished a task. The child may have dissociated or become frozen with fear of being publicly shamed, which stops them being able to achieve what they want to demonstrate. The shame of what has happened to them now threatens to come back and remind them of the traumatic experience.
- Making others look at the child who is being told off. The feeling of the eyes of others who are now staring at them can exacerbate the feelings of pain, distress and being the bad child. All difficult conversations should happen carefully and gently, assuming the child wants to please the adults.

## Boundaries in physical spaces

Boundaries can assist in a child feeling safe because they don't have to worry about feeling violated or invaded and being powerless to defend themselves. For example, if a child is sharing a bedroom, do they have a box, a cupboard, a drawer that no one else is allowed to open, so they can keep anything special or private in it? As a child grows older, they increasingly need some space where they feel they have privacy. It could be that they need somewhere to put a journal, some drawings or a teddy bear that they don't want their friends to find as they feel embarrassed but which is special to them. They need some space or a system where they can collect items that hold memories which won't be sifted through or thrown away by someone who doesn't understand their meaning. A pile of tickets or cards may look like rubbish to you but could be memories of an important or special time for them. Article 16 of the United Nations Convention on the Rights of the Child (United Nations, 1989) makes it clear that children and young people have the right to privacy, just as adults do. They need to be able to exert their own rights to hold on to some meaningful things and would probably appreciate any systems to keep them organized or tidy.

It's also worth thinking about whether they have privacy for their underwear or sanitary products or they feel that no space belongs to them and therefore they have no ownership over anything. It is vital that we give children a sense of increasing power over small spaces where they can hold their own boundaries and that we don't minimalize that or be condescending towards it. We need them to grow up learning that holding their own boundaries over their body and their property is important and their own right. When adults don't respect the child's property, drawers or cupboard space, or their privacy or ability to develop their own boundaries, it is not surprising that other adults or peers don't respect the child, and then they feel unable to protect their own rights. They need to practise with adults and grow in strength and boldness to defend their own rights.

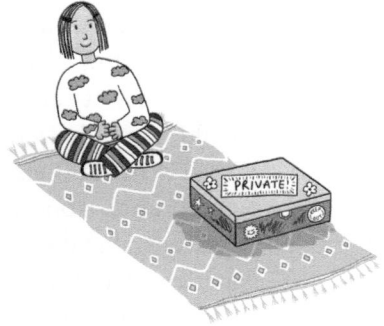

## Beauty can bring a natural calm

Art and beautiful things can be soothing to the distressed person. There have been research studies that show that people get better faster with beautiful art in hospitals. The white blank walls can be depressing and feel clinical and unhomely, but beauty can bring a sense of life and warmth which can help facilitate healing. One study found that:

> visual stimulation of nature, natural lighting, artwork, relaxing colours, and therapeutic sound can greatly accelerate the therapeutic process and create a less stressful hospital premises... [A]rtwork and natural daylight have the potentials to facilitate better healing condition on patients' wellbeing and hospital care providers' task satisfaction. (Iyendo Jnr & Alibaba, 2014)

It is important to reflect on the environment and what could be altered to enable a child to relax and feel comfortable. Some trauma-informed classrooms are abandoning the idea of clusters of tables with wall displays and bright central lights and are instead exploring classrooms with different seating styles from little sofas to floor carpets to beanbags with side lamps, and darker spaces for time to decompress. These spaces are being evaluated as I write, and the current feedback is that children find them less overstimulating and calmer as they have choice about where to work, which facilitates that sense of power when there is so much powerlessness.

A room with a fresh bunch of flowers brings a sense of life. A newly painted room with a fresh colour can feel like a brand-new start. A tidy-up of some of the clutter or a new organizing system of different boxes that can be painted so children can find what they are looking for with ease can help bring calm. All these things can make such a difference to the environment and change the stress response system of a child so that they can downregulate and feel calmer.

'The only place I felt safe was in the art room at school. The art teacher never asked me anything, but I think she just knew I needed the space to just "be". I was able to sometimes just sit quietly and feel the relief of the space. I'll always be grateful that she just let me sit there.' *James, aged 17*

## Emotionally safe

This is a vital element of feeling safe, as we explored in the last chapter about relationships. This will be considered further in the next chapter because it is as important as environmental safety.

## Conclusion

When we invite the children to consider what helps them to feel safe in the environment, they are able to share some thoughts that may surprise us! It can be surprising to find that changes such as creating a small space that the child is able to know is their own, and where they can keep some special things that help them feel safe, can bring a sense of calm to their emotions and behaviour. A beautiful, comfortable, organized space with calming smells, sounds and boundaries can enable a child to experience environmental and emotional safety. This is a foundational stage for the long-term trauma recovery journey.

## Questions to reflect on
### For parents/carers/therapeutic mentors

- Does this child have a space they prefer to be in? What is it like?
- Do they seem unsettled in any specific space? What is that like?
- Do they seem to be sensorily sensitive to noise, sight, smell or touch? What could help others to know about making the child feel more environmentally safe?
- Does the child have any specific items or ways of feeling comforted? Music, touch, smell, texture?
- What kind of environment seems to be important to avoid? Can you prepare the child for that space by providing comfort or methods to enable a sense of felt safety? (For example, a dentist visit could be scary but a teddy/physical comfort/music and a promise of a milkshake afterwards could make it bearable.)
- Does the child have a sense of privacy and boundary over an area, a drawer, a space that is for their eyes only where they can practise holding their own boundary and no one will mock them or push down the boundary?

### For therapists

- How do you manage risk assessments and health and safety within the space you use?
- How have you created a space to work in which feels sensorily safe and secure? Have you thought about the doors, windows, walls and sensory aspects of the room giving signals of safety and comfort?

# CHAPTER 5

# Emotional Safety

## Safety as a foundation to trauma recovery

It is quite clear that a child cannot begin to recover from trauma or process the past trauma memories until they feel that they are safe from those who may hurt them. They may need reassurance that they won't be left undefended if another terrifying experience occurs. Therefore, for trauma recovery to be facilitated, the foundations that need to be laid are safety and stabilization. Physical safety is vital because the child will otherwise be unable to come out of the fight, flight, freeze, flop, fawn reactions because it would be dangerous for them to do so. When physical safety has been established as far as we are able to and the child doesn't face further abuse, bullying, neglect or terror, then building emotional safety needs to be the primary focus. However, it is not just about physical safety because 'it is not enough for a child to be safe – they need to feel safe – and it's not enough for a child to be secure – they need to feel secure' (de Thierry, 2019, p.47).

It can seem ironic and painful for those who are seeking help that emotional safety is a vital foundation that everything else needs to be built on, as this can feel like a mountain to climb for already exhausted and traumatized people. Both the traumatized child and those around them are usually significantly impacted by the chaos and volatility that are the consequences of surviving the traumatic experiences. The immediate and developing survival and defence mechanisms that are automatic and often necessary can cause an increase in instability and exhaustion. This chapter will aim to explore how to help a child or young person find enough of a sense of felt safety so that trauma recovery can be made possible, because without safety, the child is unable to turn off their defensive mechanisms and learn or think or laugh. We know that 'a person will think, learn, feel, and behave differently when they are afraid compared to when they feel safe' (Perry & Winfrey, 2022, p.89).

## Feeling emotionally safe is about relationships

For a child to feel emotionally safe, it is mostly about them having access to a consistent relationship that facilitates a sense of calm and comfort. A child begins to feel emotionally safe if they have an available adult who is kind, predictable and helpful.

Emotional safety is vital because it enables the child to be able to explore and notice the areas that have been impacted by the trauma, the possible defence mechanisms, the thinking that has got muddled and the beliefs about the world that may be distorted. Exploring such areas is impossible if they still feel terrified, powerless and afraid of adults and are stuck in assuming the worst about everyone around them. When a child is stuck in defending themselves and surviving, they are unable to suddenly stop doing that and trust us! It takes repetitive positive experiences with a kind adult over a long period of time for them to begin to relax and share some of their feelings, stories and muddles.

When the children can express something that is not easy to share because it feels vulnerable, and the adult's response is one that does not minimalize, tease, shame or ignore the words but instead shows compassion, kindness and empathy but not in too intense a way, then they may begin to lose that automatic defensiveness or fast withdrawal or avoidance and may instead slowly begin to trust. Porges (2011) explains that 'the neuroception of familiar individuals and individuals with appropriately prosodic voices and warm, expressive faces translates into a social interaction promoting a sense of safety in most individuals' (p.58).

The challenge is that unless the child feels able to explore those vulnerable feelings and muddles, they cannot easily have access to the part of their brain that enables them to think, reflect and be rational and reasonable because they are stuck in survival behaviours.

Every child should be given the opportunity to find safety, both externally and internally, and should not have to layer on protective behaviours as they grow.

When a child cannot find that safety in a warm, consistent, nurturing, kind, relationship – which could be for all sorts of reasons, such as if the parent was also traumatized or ill, or if they were not able to be physically or emotionally present or if they were the source of the terror – then the child internalizes all these big experiences and they begin to fester and rumble. (de Thierry, 2020, p.90)

As adults, we have to be intentional about helping them feel that there is enough space for them to express and explore feelings and experiences that didn't feel 'that good', so that they can begin to learn how to reflect on why that could have been their experience.

We also need to be aware of the levels of emotional energy each child has at any given point, because we recognize that when a child's 'muddy buckets' are already feeling 'full', then they will have less capacity for any challenges and asking them to do something demanding is like lighting a match near petrol!

## What does safety feel like?

Safety should feel the opposite of scary, unsettling, distressing or upsetting. It should feel comfy, predictable, contained, and the child should feel able to express who they are and what they think without fear of causing distress.

An emotionally safe culture is one where transparency and honesty are valued, and secrets and sneaky behaviour are not colluded with.

Safety is felt in a person's nervous system, body, emotions and mind. Their body feels calm and not full of adrenaline or stress, and doesn't feel nervy or agitated or on edge. Their nervous system feels relaxed, and the person can laugh and think easily, and is not easily startled or zoned out. When they feel safe, they can easily ask questions, think and reflect naturally. They can articulate any boundaries or needs that they may have. They can feel a growing sense of confidence in using their voice and expressing emotions, opinions, thoughts and worries.

Here are some examples of how children and young people have described a safe place:

'A comfortable environment where you feel like there is trust and you can express your own opinion.' *Boy, aged 15*

'My fluffy Pig, familiarity, warmth, feeling welcome, space just for me, my parents and Nanny and Grandad.' *Girl, aged 7*

'When my body doesn't feel tense, twisted or heavy.' *Boy, aged 9*

'When people are giggling and laughing, and no one is sad or cross. I like that.' *Girl, aged 9*

'Being in my bed or playing on the trampoline.' *Boy, aged 12*

'When I am snuggled in my tent with all my blankets and a story read to me.' *Boy, aged 8*

'When I know my mum is around and can help if I need it.' *Girl, aged 14*

'When I'm in bed and I don't have to get up early or do anything.' *Boy, aged 15*

'When I can sit quietly in the art room and smell the paint and be in that creative space.' *Boy, aged 17*

'When I am with my family.' *Girl, aged 11*

'When I am reading a book and no one is shouting or angry.' *Boy, aged 12*

## Neuroception

The way we humans assess if we feel safe or not is by scanning our environment and our internal senses for signs of danger and signs of safety; this is called neuroception and interoception. I describe neuroception in my book on complex trauma and dissociation:

> It is an automatic, primitive, instinctive process where our own nervous system assesses the safety or risk around us and then instinctively reacts as a result of the evaluation. For example, if we have experienced a house fire and we go to a friend's house for fireworks night and we are

picturing fireworks in our imagination but as we arrive we smell fire, our neuroception could suggest that we are not safe and make a run from the house despite our cognitive brain knowing it will probably be a bonfire. (de Thierry, 2020, p.93)

Children consciously, subconsciously and automatically assess safety by noticing the facial expressions and tone of voice of the adults around them. They notice their body posture, how they interact with others, and the general atmosphere. They may make comments about an adult being 'okay' and 'nice', which may look as if they aren't analysing their environment, but the words don't tell the full picture! Children can have strong emotional reactions about adults they don't like, and it's important to spend time being curious about what the child is picking up on. It could be something that's important for you to know because they may not be feeling safe for good reasons, or it could be what is called 'faulty neuroception', where the child has wrongly assumed the adult is not safe because of the colour of their clothes or their accent which reminds them of a time when they weren't safe. Faulty neuroception is due to the child experiencing something unpleasant and then not being able to fully process or make sense of the feelings. Now memories which could be visual, sensory or confusing cause negative reactions that draw the conclusion that they are unsafe. For example, an adult who shouted at them for making a mistake was wearing a red jumper, and now the child has a strong reaction to an adult who isn't smiling and is wearing a red jumper. They may not be aware of the memory of the shouting adult in the past, but they have an instinctive negative reaction towards this adult who is now wearing red and they may not be able to explain why.

Children who have experienced frightening encounters with adults become hypervigilant and sensitive to the smallest shift in an adult's nervous system, facial reaction, tone of voice or clothing. They are constantly wired to search for signs of danger, change or safety. Survivors of trauma feel unsafe in their own bodies because there can be so many signals of danger that they can't bring to the conscious easily to reflect on what could be behind the panic and discomfort, until they have someone to help them. Music (2019) explores how he had to spend a lot of time playing football with a client because he 'needed an experience of safety, an absence of threat, even if this makes for uneventful therapy with too much football...he needed this before re-encountering his traumatic past' (p.120).

Children assess if it's the best time to talk to their parents or carers about something they did wrong by looking at their face, their body posture and getting a 'feel' for if it's a good time or not. Sadly, some of us adults can have a nervous system that is stuck in overwhelm due to our experience of life, or we are just constantly busy or anxious, and so when we say with our words 'you can always talk to me about anything', our 'vibe' or our nervous system can seem to contradict that, and so the child doesn't feel as if they can tell us important things. That's why it is important to be aware of our own nervous system and our own sense of wellbeing and work on our own anxiety so that we offer calm, grounded, safe adult care.

## Interoception

This is similar to neuroception but is instead the process of a person attuning to what is going on inside them and what messages these feelings may be conveying. The child may be sensitive to any feelings of hunger and misunderstand those and worry that they are dying, or they may not notice that they are hungry and then feel faint and wonder why.

So an important part of the recovery process is learning to get stronger in skills of interoception that focus on what is happening inside the body. In the interoceptive space, attention turns inward; in the words of Stephen Porges (1993), it can be thought of as our 'sixth sense'. Children need to gently and slowly be helped to have courage to be curious about their body sensations, and learn to let their internal world be seen and validated. To be able to do this, they need to have previously learned with different methods to calm themselves enough to be able to acknowledge the feeling of fear and panic without dissociating. Children need to be helped to slowly feel again because they

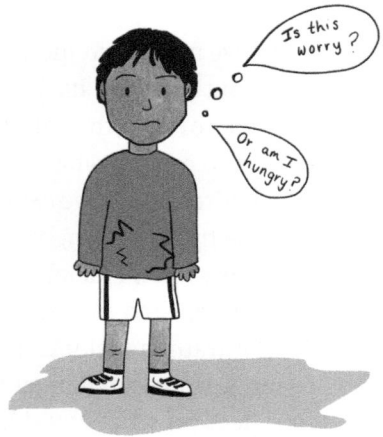

can feel deeply unsafe in their own bodies due to all that their bodies have experienced. They can often spend their lives carefully avoiding memories and flashbacks that lurk in their subconscious and bodies.

Children who experience trauma often have interrupted natural development, which can cause faulty neuroception or interoception and that can lead to other challenges such as increased anxiety or dissociation. Or they may have little confidence or practice at assessing safety or danger due to coping mechanisms that are within the freeze response, where numb, slow, lethargic reactions have been normalized. This can lead to the child not being able to assess safety or know when to stay alert and defensive and when to relax and rest. This can result inappropriate behaviour and lack of rest and play as they may be continually defensive.

## Feeling unsafe in their own skin

Some children say that they don't feel safe 'in their own skin', and that is due to either an underdeveloped interoceptive system or a faulty one, because past experiences have over-stimulated and shocked their little bodies. When a child feels like this, it is important to recognize that for them to feel safe in their own skin, they need to feel empowered to slowly feel positive sensory feelings and recognize, ponder and be less terrified of them. It does take a lot of guesswork to explore with them some experiences where they feel in control but trust enough to feel and stay feeling, without having to 'switch off those feelings'. Any shock to the body such as a medical intervention, sudden illness or some kind of traumatic violation can cause the body to feel alien to the child, and then they grow in feelings of separation towards themselves. This dissociative reaction to their body is due to it being too overwhelming for them to cope with, and so now they need to both recover from that experience and also learn to feel again.

> 'The teachers used to ask why I would stare blankly and look like I didn't care. I was just stuck. I didn't have words. I was shocked by what was happening and my body hurt, and I was struggling to believe what had happened.' *Ella, aged 16*

Shock is a sudden, terrifying and overwhelming experience that can cause a sudden intake of breath. The child may have pale skin and a rapid or shallow pulse, may exhibit disorientation and can either want to carry on as usual but look rather confused or they can't seem to move. At this point, the child needs a kind adult to gently suggest that they stay sitting or lying down for a bit and that they will stay with them until they feel able to get up. As the kind and confident adult, you could ask, 'I am wondering how your leg/arm/body feels now?' It is important not to rush the questions but follow the lead of the child for the pace of conversation. The kind, calm presence of an adult can be sufficient to help them release some of the emotions and body tension which can otherwise be stored internally long term. Sometimes a child has experienced shock, and they can continue to be shocked for some time, despite them looking more 'normal' and their breathing seeming to be less strained. Children need to be able to understand the normal shock reaction – for example, by seeing and talking about how animals react when they are scared and shocked by a loud noise, or through story books – so that they can notice these feeling responses in themselves, and learn what is a normal reaction to feeling very frightened. Once they can notice this themselves, they can learn to find healthy mechanisms to help their body and brain know that they are safe and can move to safety.

Van der Kolk explains the impact of war experiences of frontline soldiers, which summarizes how children can feel as a result of trauma:

> I am aware that I, without realizing it, have lost my feelings – I don't belong here anymore, I live in an alien world. I prefer to be left alone, not disturbed by anybody. They talk too much – I can't relate to them – the only busy themselves with superficial things. (van der Kolk, 2014, p.186)

## When the trusted adult is not around

Some adults believe that it can be unhealthy for a child to depend on or need an adult, and they can assert that it is important to help the child rely less on adults so that they can grow into independence. Research and experience show us that when a child has had enough consistent, emotionally available adults who care for them, they are able to grow in confidence and they begin to push away the adult they used to need to have in close proximity. A healthy attachment relationship in childhood leads the child to mature into an adult who is able to 'find the more comfortable personal path through life, valuing relationships yet independently competent' (Rees, 2007). This is a positive sign of them having enough of their needs met that they are able to come and find a safe adult when they need one but can also run off in confidence.

When an adult is not going to be physically available for the child, they can prepare a bag or box or item for the child to be a 'transitional object' that holds a reminder of their relationship and that they haven't forgotten them, that they still care but are unable to be in close proximity (Winnicott, 1953). When a parent of a young child draws a face on their child's hand or pops a little teddy in their pocket, the child can look at the drawing or hold the teddy and remember the parent who loves them. When a classroom assistant has to be away from the room, they can leave a little teddy or cushion or box of fiddle toys in a space that the child knows is for them if they need comfort. This feeling of 'being held in mind' is essential for the traumatized child who has an unconscious fear of further rejection, abandonment or loss.

## Transitioning important relationships

When we recognize that adult relationships and some peer relationships are a source of emotional safety for a child, we can then see how much focus we need to give to any changes to their availability. In a school setting, we see that a child who has a history of trauma may find transitions such as a new teacher, a temporary teacher or a friend leaving can cause big emotional and behavioural reactions, and the child may not be able to understand why they are feeling what they are feeling.

It's vital for staff of schools where a child is leaving, having been there for some time, to help them collect some memories over time and have some way of reconnecting in the future. When this change is rushed, it can cause the child to assume that nothing is forever, everything is short term and so there is no reason to 'settle' anywhere. This has implications for other factors such as relationships and even decisions they may make in the future. The subconscious thinking can be:

- This person won't be around soon anyway.
- I expect the person I like will leave/die/move class, so I won't get too attached.
- I may as well hate it here because if I love it, then it will be harder when I can't come again.
- That adult is so kind and I am scared that I may lose them and need that feeling of being cared for, so I will reject them and make it hard for them to be kind to me. That's easier than them rejecting me.

The best thing to help subconscious thinking that is impacting someone is to gently be curious about the kind of thoughts that other children have and see how they react. It is often painful for a traumatized child to hear an adult making assumptions or asking directly, 'Is this something you think?' as they will often shrug their shoulders and avoid replying because it feels too invasive and vulnerable to admit it.

## Emotional safety in peer friendships

A child who has been traumatized may also need help with friendships. The child may need assistance to navigate friendships and learning to trust others and when to get help from an adult. Some traumatized children can look as if they are in their own world due to the fear of rejection or being nervous about reading social cues that they are not familiar with. Power games often help us realize that powerlessness is a theme, which can give us an insight into some of the struggles the child may be having in other settings. Sometimes they can seem controlling or dominating due to fear of being a victim. These children need to see negotiation and taking turns modelled regularly, with clear emotional expression that is measured, so that they can be less afraid of losing out or being rejected. It is only by practising these relational skills that they gain strength, but some traumatized children don't have much opportunity to do this due to their volatility.

Children who struggle with feeling emotionally safe due to past experiences of relational trauma may not easily relax into an intuitive rhythm of relationship which other children may find natural. The ups and downs, the winning and losing, the intensely exclusive friendship and the group friendship experiences can all provoke feelings of confusion and powerlessness, which can then cause an escalation of feelings of fear or shame. Children may need some careful navigating through possible expectations of relationships, according to their age and setting.

Ultimately, a child needs to feel a sense of belonging, and when that seems to be at risk, they can present with defence mechanism to survive where they don't feel like they have 'a place'. Brené Brown (2021) describes belonging as an experience where the person feels 'accepted, included, respected in, and contributing to a setting or anticipating the likelihood of developing this feeling' (p.165). When someone doesn't feel as if they belong in a home, a school, a friendship group or another space, they can conclude that it is because there is something wrong with them and so they can then expect that in other settings.

## Reasons why feeling safe could be a challenge for traumatized people

- A relationship/therapeutic regular session is strictly limited to six or ten weeks for Type II or III trauma. The possible loss at the end means that they may struggle to really engage because the probability of feeling rejected and abandoned is too high.
- An environment feels dehumanizing, such as settings with access restrictions to water and toilets.
- An environment uses shaming or humiliation to make children conform.
- An environment where 100% attendance is rewarded. Absence for many reasons such as medical challenges and sickness can be unavoidable, and no one should be punished for those.
- Spaces and places have over-simplified trauma recovery and expectations that cause pressure to please the adults.
- Provisions focus on thresholds and often people find that they are too unstable or not unstable enough to access the support they need.
- There seem to be no boundaries in spaces with lots of children and other children could cause chaos and threats.
- Adults are anxious, stressed, overwhelmed, defensive or angry.
- We don't recognize that to be vulnerable is a risk and costs us all,

but to avoid vulnerability creates isolation and defence mechanisms that confuse us.
- A child has to come to a family meeting with those adults who have hurt them or not protected them, so they are unable to talk about that or disclose what happened.

We know that when humans feel safe, we can laugh, think, create and be vulnerable, which leads to stronger relationships. We also know that when we are in a survival state the neural activity is primarily found in the brainstem (primitive, automatic) and limbic (relational, emotional) area of the brain, which means that there is significantly less neural activity in the prefrontal cortex where thinking, reflection, empathy, negotiation, imagination and creativity take place. Fear can cause us to be more comfortable with a daily routine that requires little cognitive effort and can be achieved with instinctive automatic behaviour, because our brain can be taken up with trying to survive. (de Thierry, 2021, p.35)

## Conclusion

Emotional safety is a vital foundation that needs to be focused on and built. It isn't a stage and process that starts and ends, but something that each person needs to be familiar with for the rest of their life. They need to be able to answer the question, 'How do I feel safe?'

The key areas to consider are the child's relationships and how permanent or transient they are, along with how the child is currently assessing danger or safety.

## Questions to reflect on to help assess how they are finding safety
For parents/carers/therapeutic mentors

- Is this child currently as physically and emotionally safe as you are able to help them to be?
- What could you do to increase their feeling of safety?
- Who do they feel emotionally safe with? Which adults and friends?

- What transitions may be coming up and how can they be sensitively navigated (for example, a new school year or teacher, a change of home/school/club)?
- What signs of safety does your child notice more than others (for example, facial reactions, smells, a sensory comfort, a friendly person or a familiar person)?
- What does your child see as a sign of danger which they may have an exaggerated reaction towards (for example, an angry face, a bored face, noisy people or silence)?
- What would your child list as things that make them feel emotionally safe and how can these be strengthened or shifted to be more appropriate for different settings?

## For therapists

- What do you do to create safety in the sessions?
- How do you assess how safe the child feels and enable them to feel able to explore the feelings of whatever may threaten their sense of safety?
- How do you work with children in the short term, knowing that they may be beginning to trust you now and the end may cause a rupture to that positive experience? How do you ensure that they don't feel shame and are further distressed?

# CHAPTER 6

# Healthy Habits

Trauma can impact many aspects of a child's life, and as an adult taking the role of supporting a child towards recovery, it's important to recognize that the journey is a slow and steady move from surviving each day to seeing signs and sparks of hopeful change. In this mindset, it's important to recognize that there are some vital elements that can help everyone make positive progress, and one of those is to focus a little bit on building some healthy habits and normal rhythms. When each day is focused on just trying to survive the turbulence and chaos of trauma symptoms, issues like food and exercise can seem irrelevant and just add further feelings of shame or fear. However, when tiny changes can be facilitated, they can be a positive foundation for the trauma recovery work and can be fuelled by an intentional refusal to be destroyed by the trauma.

## The importance of sleep

Many people of all ages can find that sleep is impacted by trauma. They can find themselves restless at night, avoiding bedtime, or they may be able to articulate that the possibility of nightmares, flashbacks or memories being processed in some way can cause a fear of bedtime. All these are difficult realities, but when we can recognize the essential elements of a good night's sleep, we can be more intentional about learning how to overcome some of the challenges that seem to interrupt it. Sleep is more important than just avoiding the unpleasant feeling of being tired the next day; it is a process which enables the repair of muscles, tissues and bone and aids healthy growth and memory processing. Sleep can also decrease the child's irritability, anxiety, depression, emotional dysregulation and general feelings of hopelessness.

A team in the USA conducted a research project with 12,000 children aged 9 and 10 to see how lack of sleep affects brain structure and other outcomes. The researchers found that children with fewer than nine hours of sleep had more mental health and behavioural challenges than those who got sufficient sleep. The impact included the following list of symptoms of lack of sleep: 'impulsivity, stress, depression, anxiety, aggressive behaviour, and thinking problems'.

The research continued:

> The children with insufficient sleep also had impaired cognitive functions such as decision making, conflict solving, working memory, and learning. Differences between the groups persisted at the two-year follow-up. Children who had insufficient sleep – less than nine hours per night – at the beginning of the study had less grey matter or smaller volume in certain areas of the brain responsible for attention, memory, and inhibition control, compared to those with healthy sleep habits, these differences persisted after two years, a concerning finding that suggests long-term harm for those who do not get enough sleep. (Yang, Xie & Wang, 2022)

When we recognize that sleep is a priority for health and the process of recovery from trauma, it's important to work out what factors can help a child sleep better. Some of those factors could be connected to changes needed regarding diet, exercise, time in nature and less screen time. Research suggests that when we exercise more and have longer time spent outside, we sleep better.

> There is strong evidence supporting the associations between daily physical activity and sleep parameters not only in the adult population but also in children and adolescents. Moreover, reduced physical activity and increased screen time have been shown to adversely impact older children's sleep. Indeed, that study showed that physical activity and outdoor play specifically were favourably associated with most sleep outcomes in toddlers and preschoolers. (Larrinaga-Undabarrena *et al.*, 2023)

It's easy to recognize that in an era before screens, where children played outside for hours and walked more than they got lifts in cars, children did sleep better. Regular bedtimes and a routine to prepare for bed, including self-care and comforting experiences, are also helpful for the child to feel ready for bed. Often a child needs to process some of the day's experiences before bed, and if they can't do that easily, it can cause them to feel too restless to fall asleep easily – so if you are the parent or carer helping a child to get ready for sleep, make sure you've made some time for them to tell you anything that they need to tell you in order to make sense of it.

Bedtime routines can help aid easier sleep. Cleaning teeth and washing, reading together, a warm drink and some calming stories or sounds can help the child feel less scared and more supported. Some children need to be patted or stroked as if they were a tiny baby; this helps them feel more secure and able to drift into the comfort of sleep with less fear.

For sleep to be less stressful, it is helpful to avoid caffeinated drinks, limit screen brightness and introduce muscle relaxation exercises alongside some breathing exercises so that the child can slowly feel their body relax into sleep.

## Food and diet

When families are trying to survive trauma, and staying alive and functioning is the goal, any additional demand or expectation can feel overwhelming. Fast food and premade food are the easiest option for sustenance, and when battling through emotional explosions and new symptoms of distress that are impacting others as well, they can seem to be the only option if just getting up in the morning is a challenge. However, when food is understood to be the fuel that enables the child to develop a healthy brain and body which can enable trauma to be processed with more energy, it becomes vital to learn some solutions to the challenge of eating healthily while feeling overwhelmed. Healthy food can also help sustain clear thinking and energy to keep co-regulating with the distressed child.

> The foods we eat provide the construction materials we need to build healthy resilient brain cells and the fuel we need to energize them. If we don't eat the right foods, none of our cells will develop or function properly, and any number of things can and will go wrong – including

many things no medication can address. Medications can and do change brain chemistry, and they have their place, but I'm convinced that the most powerful way to change brain chemistry is through food, because that's where brain chemicals come from in the first place… Optimal mental health requires that your whole brain be made of the right stuff. (Ede, 2024, p.19)

Poverty or the cost-of-living crisis can certainly lead to assumptions that a healthy diet is a more expensive diet. However, there are ways to shop and cook that are not exhausting or demanding but which can facilitate healing and sustenance to the whole family where it becomes an intentional choice to work at recovering from the trauma that has been inflicted.

## Hygiene and caring for themselves

It is recognized that when people begin to struggle with life and find it overwhelming, one of the first things that can become compromised is their ability to look after themselves. Therefore, as adults caring for children, we must make sure that we teach them in a relational, caring way how important it is for them to keep themselves clean. When a child can be aware of and want to have clean clothes, when they want to wash regularly, clean their teeth and care for their hair, they are less likely to add additional struggle to their friendships. Friendships are vital, and children are quick to notice and tease children who are not showing care about their own appearance. The important element is that it is taught in a warm, caring way that reduces shame rather than causing increased shame. It is also vital that the issue does not become a place where control or domination is exerted, because that always causes a breakdown in relational connection.

## Screen time versus play time

As a parent myself, I do recognize children's reliance on screens for connecting with peers and finding out all the useful (and less useful) things that a young person may be curious about. However, I think we all also know how damaging it can be when a child is very dependent on screens and is losing the ability to differentiate between fact and opinion, fantasy and reality, friend and abuser, truth and lie. We need to be active in emotionally connecting with the children in our worlds, where they feel able to ask questions or to reflect with us if there was something they saw that they are not sure what to do with.

We recognize that children who play and explore the world they live in are healthier and can develop skills that are essential for a life filled with positive relationships and activities.

The screen can feel like a safety blanket to a child who has had relational trauma or been bullied or teased or let down by others as it feels more stable and consistent and therefore less risky. Screens can also cause significant anxiety, and the child can be concerned about not knowing the latest joke or meme, so they need us to help guide them into a confidence that is not dependant on always knowing the latest popular social media post. I know that's easier said than done, but the most effective way is not only to limit time on screens but to fill up their time with other more meaningful activities.

## COVID impact on playing

Playing with friends is vital for younger children and important for all ages of child. Since COVID and the lock-in months that many children were exposed to, where their relational interactions and sensory experiences were significantly limited, many children seem to be displaying some behaviours which may have been viewed as developmentally delayed. Several studies show negative psychological effects on children and families as a result of the pandemic (Brooks *et al.*, 2020; Loades *et al.*, 2020; Panchal *et al.*, 2021). It's important that we recognize that children develop skills in a use-dependent way, and so when they were unable to have the repetitive experiences required to develop many of the social skills such as sharing or negotiating or turn taking, they may appear to be delayed but in fact just need more experiences to practise and learn.

The United Nations Convention on the Rights of the Child (United Nations, 1989) explains the rights of all children and teenagers. It states that 'every child has the right to play – whoever they are, wherever they live and whatever they believe'. This recognition of the central aspect that play should have in a child's life as they seek to make sense of the world is foundational.

Playing is essential for healthy children to develop skills that are needed for imagination and creativity, relationship skills and physical skills, and it helps them solve problems and work out how things work. It is a way for children to grow in their physical, emotional, relational and mental development.

Children who have experienced trauma may be less confident in their play as they may feel nervous about taking the lead or feeling controlled (Nicholson, 2020; Brown, 2014). They may struggle to share ideas or feel stupid if they are asked and cannot think straight because of the fear of rejection or failure. Traumatized children can struggle to take turns or share because they can feel anxious about being left out or people being unkind to them, as that has often been their experience. Creating emotionally safe play opportunities is vital for children of all ages. As they get older, they learn to be more specific about what they enjoy and are interested in and what they would rather avoid, but opportunities to play, create, try something new and practise some relational and creative challenges can be scary but also confidence building when they go well.

## Exercise and fitness

For some children who have experienced trauma, the shock and horror of what has happened can be so overwhelming that they demonstrate an overactive fight response with strong defensive behaviours that can lead to sudden agitated actions. They may be hypervigilant, jumpy, angry or controlling so that they don't have the feeling of powerlessness. Other children may instead have a more exaggerated startle response, or they may run down the corridor or walk out of the classroom at the slightest hint of conflict or terror. These children may find any form of exercise helpful and a source of relief compared to sitting still. It's a way to discharge some of the agitation and nervous energy and enables them to concentrate afterwards when they enjoy the feelings of post-exercise relief.

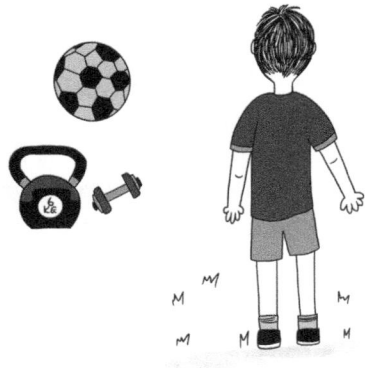

Some children, however, may instead freeze and stare blankly, look as if they don't care, zone out or act lethargic, or complain of being tired a lot. Those children who are more prone to a freeze response may find the concept of exercise difficult and may avoid, refuse or complain as they even seem to struggle to move from classroom to home. They would rather sit still or, better still, lie down. They are exhausted from surviving the levels of emotional reactivity or internal turmoil which are hidden inside them, away from others' ability to see. For these children, exercise seems to be entirely cruel, and they need to understand more about their body and how it works to be able to comprehend the thought of it. These traumatized children are instinctively trying to reserve their energy to stay alive, and so unless it is explained gently to them how their bodies can become stronger and healthier, they generally won't comply. When they are slowly able to be helped to feel their own heartbeat without wincing or being scared, and when they can learn about breathing and listen to their breath, they can begin to befriend their bodies. This is the first starting point of engaging with exercise. They need to understand more about their bodies, have their fears reduced of being further hurt, know how to listen to what their body is communicating and then exert their own boundaries.

Exercise is vital for healthy living, but it needs to be approached through the relational lens that is curious about what the child has experienced and therefore what fears they may have that they cannot yet express, and so instead they use avoidance or anger as a shield to defend themselves. Research has found that 'physical fitness was significantly and positively associated with children's mental health. Additionally, children with higher-level physical fitness reported greater resilience and lower-level anxiety, which in turn contributed to their mental health' (Li *et al.*, 2022).

It would be ideal if every child was able to find a sport or active hobby that they enjoy in childhood and could continue to enjoy as they grow older, where they are intentional about looking after their body and having fun.

'I used to be scared of exercise because it made my heart beat faster and harder and so I thought I was going to die. The only other time I felt like that was when I was being beaten up so I didn't understand why other children used to like running. It scared me. I get it now and it can feel good.' *Sam, aged 11*

## Learning and school

When a child has experienced trauma, there are neurobiological changes that occur which can make learning challenging. The part of the brain responsible for thinking, processing, reflecting and learning is not easily accessible when the part of the brain that is wired to survive is fully alert and scanning for danger. A traumatized child can struggle with the motivation to learn, the ability to reflect or be curious, the relationships in a group of children and the routine or lack of routine that schools can offer. A large collaboration of professionals researched the impact of trauma on learning and acknowledged that:

> Trauma can impair learning. Single exposure to traumatic events may cause jumpiness, intrusive thoughts, interrupted sleep and nightmares, anger and moodiness, and/or social withdrawal – any of which can interfere with concentration and memory. (National Child Traumatic Stress Network, 2008)

For children who have experienced trauma, the expectations that need to be met can be difficult because the possibility of shame, rejection, failure and isolation can be terrifying. It is important for the school to be a place that understands the impact of trauma and can know a little of the triggers or sensitivities that the child may have. A trauma-informed culture is not one where everyone can do what they like without boundaries or consequences, but it is a culture that understands that behaviour is often communication, that distressed children have symptoms of distress that can be decreased when they feel safer and that relationships are key to children feeling safe.

These days, however, in many education settings, because they are struggling with reduced finances and increased numbers of children who need individualized plans, it can be challenging to be able to provide what many of them would love to be able to do. It is therefore imperative to try and work as collaboratively as possible with the school staff as they try their best to provide what is increasingly impossible to do for each child.

Wanting to learn and being curious about the world are a sign of a healthy brain and child. When that curiosity and fascination about the world is declining, we must do what we can to rekindle the love of learning. If these children have survived so much trauma that they are now mostly functioning in an automatic state of survival, then it can take time for them to be curious about anything more than why others seem to be doing things that seem entirely pointless. These children have been robbed of the joy and adventure of learning, and they need to be able to feel safer before they can move on from their hypervigilance and defensive coping mechanisms and explore anything other than how to stay alive.

It is important that the child can have their natural interests incubated and that each child is able to be seen, heard and celebrated for the unique character that they are. When a home or youth club or other similar setting can model an interest or fascination in certain subjects, and they can watch to see what seems to cause a spark of interest in the child, they can then aim to help them grow in knowledge. This develops the skills of learning and so the subject matter isn't that important; the learning process and excitement about facts and knowledge collection is an experience that is foundational for a love of learning to be nurtured. Children can become obsessed with rocks, dinosaurs, the latest cartoon character or football star. It doesn't matter what the subject matter is; what matters is their ability to experience the fun of growing in knowledge.

It is important that children understand that everyone is unique, and each child is meant to be different from other children. Their uniqueness is something that should be celebrated by those who love them, and no one should tease or laugh at anyone else.

## Conclusion

When a child has been traumatized, daily life can be full of challenging experiences which can lead to the family only managing to focus on surviving day to day. Healthy habits can seem impossible or irrelevant to a family in crisis or ongoing stress, and yet we recognize that when these areas of a child's life such as sleep, diet, exercise, hobbies and play can be reflected on and strategies implemented, recovery can be easier. Healthy habits provide a strong foundation for a child to recover from trauma.

## Questions to reflect on
### For parents/carers/therapeutic mentors

- How is the sleep of the child you are thinking about? Is there anything specific that you could begin to introduce to improve the duration and quality of sleep?
- How is the diet and nutrition of the child? Is there a way to introduce a wider range of nutritionally dense foods?
- How is the child spending their time? How long do they have on screens and how could you decrease that without it negatively impacting your relationship?
- How do they currently play? What is their favourite activity to play? What were their early play experiences like when they were under 5 years old? Do they need to experience some play that they missed out on in those developing years?
- Does this child enjoy exercise? What happens when you suggest some? Do they understand some of the biological reasons for moving and exercising?
- What is their learning approach? Are they curious about the world or are they stuck in survival? What topics have they shown interest in? Could you rekindle a learning journey for them?

### For therapists

- Have you spent time exploring what COVID was like for this child and how it may have impacted their development?
- What could you do to support the adults to help them with these habits while they are also spending energy and time building positive relationships with the children?

# CHAPTER 7

# What Does a Trauma Recovery Journey Look Like?

## The first stage: starting the journey

One of the hardest stages of the journey can be acknowledging the child's distress and finding enough emotional energy to be vulnerable and have hope that things can change. It can be tough as the parent or carer of the child to acknowledge how things are, and it can feel unfair that there have been some life experiences for the child you are supporting that have been unavoidable and have caused damage, and that many of their behavioural and emotional challenges could be due to that. Reading this book can be a big leap into a new way of thinking and reflecting on the concept that our brains are malleable and adaptable and that change and recovery are possible. It's important here to keep remembering that most of us have tried our best with what we had available to us – the knowledge, emotional courage and energy – but now we can dive into this journey and be the best supporter, champion and encourager that we can be to help children recover from what has impacted them so deeply. Brené Brown (2021) praises all who are trying to approach trauma recovery with a mindset of humility and describes it as 'openness to new learning combined with a balanced and accurate assessment of our contributions, including our strengths, imperfections, and opportunities for growth' (p.245).

Trauma can be a difficult topic to talk and think about unless it is about someone else's life! It takes courage and energy to reflect and wonder where things may have gone wrong in our own lives or in the lives of those we care about. Denial is a strong culture that normalizes the 'lack of tolerance for the emotional vulnerability that traumatized people experience. Little time is allotted for the working through of emotional events' (Levine, 1997, p.48). This book that you are reading explores how unhelpful and damaging that can be for all ages.

Trauma recovery is possible, but it isn't always easy because the very nature of trauma is the deep feeling of the threat of life and death that is intertwined through the nervous system, body, emotions, subconscious, memories and relationships. The human brain and body adapt to enable survival in the face of an experience that is threatening to our lives and to our ability to survive. Those changes are complex and the healing and transforming 'back' to 'normal' isn't a linear journey. It isn't always something that is clearly visible because the changes and positive moves forward are often in tiny steps that need repeating many times, which eventually makes the changes visible. When a person begins to realize on a deeper level that what happened to them was trauma, was unjust, was wrong and not their fault, they may begin to have memories of fragments of their story that can interrupt their daily life. These can be flashbacks, body memories or emotional reactions, and the child can sometimes want to control or make sense of them or order them. It can be destabilizing for them to focus on these memories because they are overwhelming and too much to cope with, which is why they became fragmented in some way. When and if they seem to become increasingly vivid and interruptive, it is usually best for the child to find some practical comfort methods and be encouraged not to dwell on what happened to them but to focus on looking after themselves now. Each child needs to have some 'anchor points', ways that they feel familiar with to quickly help them feel safe and comfortable when they feel as if the memories and story are becoming too storm-like on their insides. When the child is able to have therapy, they can then process the memories until they feel less overwhelming.

## It isn't as fast and as simple as learning your times tables!

The very nature of life-threatening experiences – or what the person perceived was life threatening because of their age – means that the focus from the body, brain and unconscious is to make sure that it never happens again. Ultimately, the traumatized person is now wired to make sure that when a threat seems to be a possibility, there is enough energy to stay alert and be ready to fight that threat. Previously terrifying situations become memories that act as reminders and warnings in flashbacks, nightmares and triggers, causing the person to stay hyperaroused and ready for the danger, because to relax or feel calm would be a danger to life. That is how traumatized people become wired to stay alive in the face of so much danger in the world – because there are so many humans who could be dangerous and cause hurt. Perry and Winfrey (2021) explain how our society can often misunderstand the child's response to trauma and the disruption it can cause for them. What is:

> adaptive for children living in chaotic, violent, trauma-permeated environments becomes maladaptive in other environments, especially school. The hypervigilance of the Alert state is mistaken for ADHD [attention deficit hyperactivity disorder]; the resistance and defiance of Alarm and Fear get labelled as oppositional defiant disorder; flight behaviour gets them suspended from school; fight behaviour gets them charged with assault. The pervasive misunderstanding of trauma-related behaviour has a profound effect on our educational, mental health, and juvenile justice systems. (p.92)

*The impact of trauma is on many levels, which all need undoing and redoing and then strengthening.* It is easier for the child who has been traumatized to heal and recover while they are still children because the brain is still developing; while it is so malleable, it can change with more ease than when they become adults. It's just like learning to ride a bike or speaking another language; it's so much easier to adapt and learn such complex skills when the child is young because it takes far more neural repetitions for an adult to learn the same thing compared to a child. Sadly, that's why six-week counselling or mentoring sessions aren't always going to help a child long term when they have experienced trauma. In fact, they could cause more harm if the child enjoyed the mentor's company and then they are told that they can't see them again. That can feel like additional loss for them to have to process, and so with Type II or III trauma it is not at all 'better than nothing' but in fact damaging to the already damaged understanding of relationships.

## The journey requires hard work from all involved

Ideally, many of us would love a ten-step programme that we could do for our child while eating our breakfast. Even better still, I think most of us want to just show up somewhere and have them sort us all out while we either sleep or watch a film. Young people often seem to want to know why they must be involved in the process of recovery and, worse still, why they have to work so hard and put effort in when it was never their fault in the first place. That feels like the biggest injustice of all. None of them chose what happened to them and now no one else can do most of the hard work, they must do it themselves. That feels cruel.

But as adults, if we can support them, remind them of how far they have come and simplify the wiggly path with some clear signposts, then they can be motivated and committed. The child needs to know it's worth it. When they are young, the therapy and most of the methods of healing are play based, which results in the child even enjoying some aspects of the recovery journey. They are getting some of their needs met and they can enjoy the attention, the emotional connection and the time spent with kind adults. Young people, however, usually want to choose how to spend their time and who with, and they can feel less enthralled to have to add another demand to their life, such as therapy and therapeutic care. It can sometimes seem to just add more pressure to them unless they have acknowledged the deep sadness and devastation of how their trauma symptoms have caused further pain and turmoil.

## The journey is wiggly

The trauma recovery journey is not a straight line, and sometimes along the path it can feel as if things are getting worse, but that is just a wiggle before they get better. I like to think it can be a bit like a diet – one day you are eating healthily and doing all the exercises you want to and the next day you are craving that doughnut and don't want to move. If the doughnut day was only one or two days in the month, then the progress will be fantastic, and they were just wiggles in the path that is going in the right direction.

Remember that all the behaviour we see has a reason somewhere. Children want to fit in, be accepted, play and learn, and enjoy adults being pleased with them, and they can feel trapped in behaviour that they don't understand. For example, sometimes children may confuse us because they seem to almost want to get into trouble, but there is a good reason for that.

> The children and adults we work with are so used to chaos, they actually feel more comfortable when its chaotic than when its calm... I have teachers and foster parents tell me, 'He almost acts like he wants to get punished.' And to a certain extent they are right. He is seeking a predictable response from the world. (Perry & Winfrey, 2021, p.181)

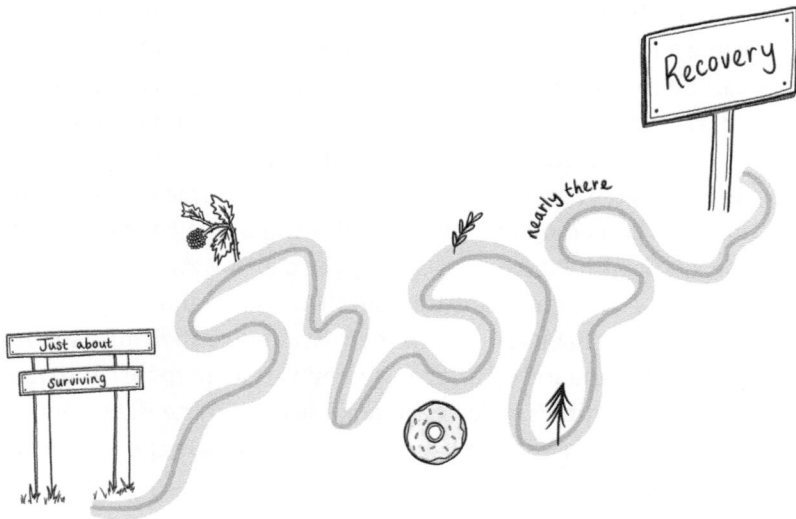

The important thing on the 'doughnut days', or the days when it seems to be getting worse, is to help the child:

- remember how far they have come
- think and maybe look at photos of some good days or activities or moments that they have had
- have some clear goals of things that they want to be able to see happen that are too difficult now, but can be achievable when there is more recovery (make sure they are specific)
- carve some time out to enable them to do things that provide comfort and where there are no emotional or physical demands on them

- focus on making sure they can feel safe, and can eat, drink and sleep.

## Remember to try and keep track of things

Sometimes it can be hard to know if you are seeing any progress in the child and therefore it can feel disheartening. The changes are usually small and sometimes even packaged in frustrating behaviours. It could be that some children may start to tease you, which may be a sign that they feel they can trust you not to be angry. It could be that the child who used to avoid all adults is now clingy towards you, which can be frustrating but could be a sign that they have formed a positive attachment to you. It's difficult to celebrate any small wins when you can't remember them! So it is important to work out some way of keeping a record of the journey. It doesn't have to be thorough or written essay each day, but a note of the dominant moods displayed, the worst points and the highlights would be enormously helpful for you to read back and see how far they and you have come.

It could be as simple as buying a cheap paper diary and writing a few words and any quick highs and lows each day. It can feel therapeutic for us as the adult to do that because it focuses us on change and drives us to see change. It can prevent us losing motivation because we are caught amid the chaos and volatility. If you really can't manage that extra thing to do each day, maybe ask a friend to have a weekly coffee with you and try and download the week's ups and downs with them so they can keep a diary for you and remind you of how far the child has come and how incredible your support has been.

The recovery journey is one that has layers and layers that need to be processed, so it is not always as simple as thinking that one area of wound is 'done' and that's it – often that's one layer of processing that wound and there may be another layer of it yet to be processed! Remember when things are tiring that researchers are clear that 'the development of the brain is an experience-dependent process; in fact, neurons and neural tissue are the most susceptible to change from experience of any tissue in the body' (Cantor et al., 2018). This means that from a neurobiological perspective, trauma recovery is possible!

## Saying sorry

One of the things that adults can avoid, because it can make things worse, is different forms of defensiveness when a child is courageous enough to share their feelings about an experience where they felt hurt. When a child is brave and honest and mentions something that the adult did that made them feel sad or upset, it can be quite destructive for the relationship if the adult reacts with shame and exclamations such as 'I am the worst adult. I knew it, I may as well give up trying.' While many adults may feel quite justified in having that feeling because they have tried their best and probably feel deeply frustrated and tired, it can stop the child and their needs becoming the focus. What the child needs is to experience an authentic apology and some time to express any specifics of what the adult could do better, along with a sense of love, acceptance and validation that they are important and them being hurt was very much unintended. When as adults we manage to regulate enough to speak and reach out with apology and care, it can move the relationship forward rather than backwards. Research (Carr, 2014) suggests that 'when modelled by a parent, an apology becomes more than just a form of conflict resolution; it is a force multiplier providing assurance of the strength within the parent-child relationship'. This research continues with assertions that saying sorry authentically to the child can impact other areas of the child's life. 'By understanding the magnitude of parental modelling of apologizing to children, it is likely that the previous correlation between prosocial behaviour and higher academic achievement may be another positive ramification of two small but powerful parental words, "I'm sorry".'

Many children have experienced adults who lie about what they have done and blame the child for things that they did wrong themselves. That's why when an adult says sorry in an authentic way about hurting them or not helping them in a way they had wanted, it can be restoring for children. No adult can avoid making mistakes, forgetting some things we have promised and sometimes getting it wrong, but we can say sorry and explain that we do not want to get it wrong. That can be healing because of the honesty and authenticity.

'When my mum said she was sorry and I felt like she meant it, I realized that she was trying her best and I actually felt a bit sorry for her. I don't think I have been that easy to parent so that helped me begin to see that she was a human too.' *Sally, aged 16*

## They will need to keep some things private

It can be hard for an adult when a child asserts their need to keep some things private. It can feel disappointing that they don't seem to trust you and won't be fully transparent with you, and it can challenge your sense of control over their journey. It is, however, important to remember that part of the journey of trauma recovery is that the child begins to explore and experiment with asking for control over some areas that they want to keep private. Healthy children who are not traumatized also explore the boundaries around secrets, where they can practise asserting boundaries and rules to help them feel safer and more in control. Traumatized children also need to exert the same power, and when that is challenged by an adult who is terrified things may go wrong, it can escalate quickly. The child may show behaviour towards you that is more synonymous with being abused or physically hit. They may scream, hit you and say they hate you. Possibly the worst consequence would be that they close down emotionally with you, withdraw and either offer you a fake style of relationship or actually develop a more compliant part of themselves to appease you while secretly remaining in control. Children need privacy and they need to be able to discuss, reflect or be heard as they practise setting boundaries around themselves. The child is not usually aware that this is a vital step of both growing up and healing from trauma because it arises from the unconscious. They don't need this process explained to them, they just need to be supported or they will feel controlled or condescended to. This boundary setting and exploration around privacy should be a positive sign of healing and restoration taking place in the unconscious if it is allowed to take place without the child feeling as if they are a chemistry experiment!

## They may change in ways you haven't predicted – hold the changes loosely

During the process of healing and recovery from trauma, the child may begin to change in ways that you haven't predicted. They often go through several changes and can change their clothes style, their sense of identity, their friendship affiliations, their favourite activities and many other areas of their life. It's important to let them have the freedom to explore who they are and how they fit into the world without affirming any specific choice but just affirming them as children who are important and valued. When an adult is too quick to validate a choice, the child can feel a sense of responsibility to appease the adult, and rather than that choice being a short phase it can become more embedded due to the relief of the validation.

It's important to hold things loosely as adults, especially around adolescence. It's also important that we explain to a child that their brain is constantly developing alongside their body growing and, therefore decisions that impact the rest of their life should be avoided until they have stopped growing and are no longer showing clear signs of distress. As adults, we know that our worst decisions are made when we are hungry or angry or distressed, and it's the same for children. Society sometimes seems to encourage children to make decisions, such as subject choices for exams, at an age when they are rarely certain what they will want to do in their adult years! We need to make sure that whatever decision children make before they get to age 24, which is approximately when the prefrontal cortex (our thinking brain) stops developing, does not have long-term impact and escalate the trauma that they have already experienced.

## They may need to have an open-door sense with professionals who have helped them

Those adults who are helpers for the child need to be available longer term to enable the child to be able to form an attachment with them that is not going to cause further attachment trauma. Short-term help can be detrimental to their experience, and it can reaffirm that only people who are paid to support them care, which doesn't feel like genuine care. This can affect their self-esteem because they can believe that they are not worthwhile and no one can 'cope with them'.

If the child does form an attachment to a therapist, teacher, teaching assistant or another adult who is nurturing to them, it would be ideal if they could have a way of being able to sense some constancy with the relationship. At the Trauma Recovery Centres (TRC®s) that I founded in 2011, we have an 'open-door policy' where the child can book in for a visit when they have left, at any time, for the rest of their life. It's lovely to see some of the children who processed some difficult experiences over many weeks or years come back and have a cup of tea and tell us their news many years later. It's not 'just a job'– it's a huge privilege to be a part of someone else's life for a few years, and as such we need to recognize the need for them to be able to have access long term, even if they don't use it.

## As the parent, try not to feel threatened when the child seems to find another adult helpful

When a child does develop an attachment with another adult, such as a sports coach, teaching assistant or therapist, try not to feel threatened by that. It could be that you have worked hard to form an attachment and it's been hard and up and down, and now you see them forming a positive attachment with another adult who you know that they are grateful for. That can be hard, but the attachment they form with a helper can enable the attachment that they are developing with you to grow stronger, especially if the helper is providing a safe place for the child to explore their feelings about you and can help them see how committed you are to their recovery. It's not in their interest to form long-term attachments with children for decades, and it is in their interest to facilitate the attachment between the child and you. When the child sees you trusting them and trusting another adult, they can feel less claustrophobic and controlled, which will strengthen your relationship.

## What about those children still living in trauma?

As Section 1 draws to a close, I am aware that some of the children you are supporting will be living in different situations where they may be stuck in a way that means it would impossible to facilitate emotional and physical safety. They could be trapped in a home that feels unsafe; they may feel powerless to change school and yet they are desperately unhappy. You may be the only adult in their life who currently has capacity to be their support, their hope and with whom they can feel safe. I have worked with adults who were traumatized as children, and they speak of the adults who did care and how they were able to keep going and have some spark of hope due to them being there. While recovery would be ideal, you are possibly in a position of being able to build the foundations of recovery through your consistent, kind, emotionally present, co-regulating, hope-filled relationship that offers safety and stability. When they are old enough to leave the current situation that is causing them the distress and overwhelm, they won't be as hopeless, but will have skills and knowledge that you have helped them develop. It's not a waste of time because you can't complete the recovery process – far from it, as these vulnerable children and young people are able to find sparks of life, hope and connection that enable them to endure relentless trauma.

I want to assure you that when you show your care and concern on your face as you listen or speak to them kindly, they internalize that look, sometimes for the rest of their lives, and it helps them believe that they are worth caring for.

Here are some things that therapeutic professionals and carers and parents can focus on:

- Building a positive relationship where they begin to trust you as an adult.
- Teaching them psychoeducation so they can understand themselves better and how their brain and nervous system work.
- Co-regulating with them so that they can begin to express emotions in a healthy way, including the emotions that they may feel each day around rejection, turmoil, sadness and anger.
- Helping them learn what brings comfort to them and what helps remind them of hope, so when they can't see you anymore, they have clear reminders that people care and have cared for them.
- Teaching them to play games and lose sometimes, share ideas with others and feel connected.
- Teaching them to care for themselves by helping them understand sleep, nutrition, exercise and the importance of finding activities that help them connect with others.
- Helping them explore their identity and what they are good at and what they would like to do when they are older.

All of these will help the child have a strong foundation to be able to process the trauma once they are safe and in a stable setting. It is life-changing work!

## What does recovery look like?

I like to think about recovery as the time when the story of what happened no longer causes physical, emotional and mental pain and where the ways to survive it are no longer coping mechanisms that stop life being lived to the full. I believe it is possible for people to know their history, be able to explain the level of pain, terror, turmoil and shock that they experienced, but know that was in the past and now they are in a different season of life. I think about the caesarean section scars I have from three of the six births of my children. I am very much aware of them, even though they hardly show and they are not impacting my life as I live day to day. However, if I do certain specific movements, I can sometimes feel a pull or a pinch that can surprise me, but the surgery was in the past and I know my body has healed from it. Trauma recovery is similar, where sometimes an experience, a sight, sound or smell may suddenly catch our breath and remind us of the past, but it doesn't cause us to have to start again on our healing journey; the scars are a sign of courage and healing.

## Conclusion

Trauma recovery is not easy, but it is worth it not only for the rest of the child's life, but also for their children who will be able to be parented in a way that changes generational trauma patterns. I hope this chapter has exposed some of the areas that can cause the path towards recovery to be a bit rocky so that you feel more equipped to be aware and steer around the bumps and rocks.

## Questions to reflect on
### For parents/carers/therapeutic mentors

- Have you noticed that some of the 'wounds' of the trauma need layers of healing? Maybe you've noticed that they seem to get better and then there is another layer?

- How have you tracked the progress made through the wiggly journey?
- Who are your support people? Where could you find some if you don't know any?
- How are you navigating the issue of privacy for the child and their need to feel power not powerlessness, while still keeping them safe?
- What other attachment figures do they have and how do you feel about them?
- What does the child look like if you imagine them no longer bothered by trauma symptoms? Picture them now!

## For therapists

- How are your systems for communication between the adult and the child? Are they comfortable for the adults and confidential, secure and recorded?
- If the child read them, would they feel cared for or would they feel betrayed?
- How are you collaborating with the primary adults and teacher to support the child?

CHAPTER 8

# The Different Ages and Application Shifts

This book is an overview of the journey towards recovery from trauma, and as such the application of the information needs to be carefully considered through the lens of the child's specific age, emotional age, current context and specific challenges. I wish I could be there to listen to each of your stories or the child's stories and help support you as you fight to get the help they deserve.

The first stage of the recovery journey that needs to be kept in focus is the creation of physical and then emotional safety for the child. This part of the journey could take several months or years of intentional work until the child is able to reflect and articulate that they feel safe and know how to help themselves feel safe. This begins to be what could be termed 'stability', because for the child there seems to be no obvious impending change or traumatic experience that they know is about to occur. When there is consistency in the child's environment because they feel seen, heard and known, and where they have built some trust, then they are ready to begin to process the trauma, heal and recover.

## Psychoeducation

All ages and children from all kinds of settings can learn about the body, the brain, the nervous system, emotions and other vital facts that enable them to feel less powerless. Children who are older usually love any YouTube videos or therapeutic story books that have been written for a younger audience as long as this is framed by explaining that you found it helpful, and you know loads of xx-year-olds (the age of child plus a few years) who have found it to be helpful even though it's aimed at little kids.

Helping children know why they behave in ways that shock them and why they struggle to sleep or have nightmares or why they sometimes can't remember something is essential to them having their dignity restored and feeling more in control of their own lives. All ages need a growing sense of knowledge about being a human, how we work best, what happens when things go wrong and how we can repair. This is another part of building a healthy foundation for recovery because it reduces shame about being a human and helps them feel more empowered on their own journey.

'I thought I was just plain bad. No one told me that the stupid things I did sometimes were because actually I was scared. Now I feel like I can prove that I'm a good kid because I understand myself better.'
*Jack, aged 9*

## Children who seem to be stuck in Type II and III trauma

I know that many of you will be reading this and be aware that the children you are supporting are unlikely to experience emotional safety or stability due to the environment that they are immersed in. Relational trauma, ongoing unrelenting poverty, transitions in primary caregivers, continual war (either domestic abuse or a military war) can all cause the child to feel as if their world is unstable and unsafe because they must navigate their way to safety each day. Can these children recover from trauma when the possibility of it still occurring is a reality? These children can certainly be helped and can have their life trajectory transformed completely by having adults supporting them while they are still living through their trauma. In Section 3, I explore the impact and recovery aspects of the different kinds of trauma experiences and how some traumas, such as abuse, need to stop before full recovery can happen, but that doesn't mean that children can't experience elements of healing and hope from having contact with positive and helpful adults while they wait for more stability and peace in their life.

When children are in long-term traumatic settings, although establishing safety and stability is usually our first aim, when that is impossible to fully guarantee, I believe it would be unethical to wait for this foundation, so instead we should help them begin to heal in different ways now, and be ready to help them recover more easily when they are able to leave those settings. Even if they have to survive traumatic settings, they can learn relational skills and emotional regulation skills, they can become aware of who they are and the defence mechanisms they use and what they are feeling, and they can begin to use emotional language to describe some of what they are coping with. These are vital and foundational aspects that can be further developed when they are old enough to access therapy that helps them to process the trauma and make a fuller recovery.

## Treatment plans

In my mind, I picture a written treatment plan to be full of feelings of hope and healing suggestions, and that's why I like the name of the plan. It should be like a small child who has a tiny scratch having warm cotton wool placed on the wound with love, compassion, care and emotional connection. We want to treat the wounds that have been made to these young lives, so that they get better. When these plans can be formed to hold and validate the child's traumatic experience and their current and possible future needs for those areas that need healing, there is hope that recovery is the primary focus.

Some plans seem to be primarily aimed at managing the symptoms which are viewed as interruptive for others and therefore need to stop, but that's not hope-filled. Each child should have an individualized 'treatment plan' which has been written reflectively and acknowledges what safe feels like for them, the trauma symptoms that need to be reduced, the attachment relationships that need strengthening and the trauma history that needs to be processed. The plan would also include how and where they could access any additional help that they would need to process and recover from trauma. All reports and plans for children would be written knowing that the child may want to read them when they are older, so the language used must reflect the care we have and the courage they are showing.

## Children aged under 5

This is the age where the brain develops at the fastest pace, and so every day or week holds the potential for positive and healthy growth and learning. In this period of a child's life, the attachment relationships are central to everything and that adult's proximity to the child is vital for positive growth. Usually, safety and stability for the young child can be significantly easier to develop because they have had fewer negative experiences that subconsciously warn them about adults being untrustworthy or scary.

Healthy habits are easier to develop in these years as they normalize good food, exercise and play rather than sugary snacks and screen time (which should be very minimal in this age group).

Environments can be more intentionally set up for the needs of the exploring baby, toddler or child so that they do not have to have a jumpy, agitated adult screaming every time the child goes towards a drawer, door or space that is not safe. Environmental safety is more obvious and it's quite instinctive to make sure things are done to avoid the child choking, swallowing poison, trapping their body or fingers, and help them stay out of danger.

Many of the traumatic events that occur in these early years can cause negative impact primarily in the child's natural development and especially their sensory processing skills. These lost developmental stages can be restored with repetitive, intentional work to 'catch up' and bring about a sense of integration. Emotional neglect is the greatest challenge to healthy development in this developmental period, and I have written a comprehensive book on how to help a child to recover from that specific trauma. The book is called *The Simple Guide to Emotional Neglect* (2023), and although the traumatic experience seems to attract less empathy, research asserts it is the most severe form of childhood trauma (Hart, Brassard & Karlson, 1996).

Children of this age are usually much more dramatic, externalized and exaggerated, which means that it is far more concerning when they are quiet, withdrawn or stare blankly or if they can't seem to be comforted or calmed down.

It is generally easier to emotionally connect in a way in which the child can feel validated, seen, heard, cared for and safe. When the adults are emotionally available enough to quickly take the time to try and help them express something of what made them feel scared or sad, and if the child can experience this repeatedly from a consistent attachment figure, they will be able to recover from trauma and grow in confidence.

Here are a few ways to help a child process something scary that has happened:

- Spend time reassuring the child that the traumatic event is now over and they are safe.
- Allow some time and space to ask them what they are thinking about what happened, in case they are muddled or worried about what they saw and heard.
- Make sure that the child doesn't see similar events happening on any screens or overhear adults discussing what happened.
- Help them use language to name some of the emotions they may have felt so that they can get familiar with those names.
- Validate their worries and fears and reassure them, comfort them and be patient with them as they process what happened. They may do this through play with their toys, which is an ideal way to help them discharge their negative emotions.

## Early trauma experiences under 5 years old

The following list shows the kind of trauma experiences or symptoms that may become apparent through an intentional assessment of the child's trauma history and would probably need an intentional trauma recovery specialist to work alongside other attachment figures to be able to facilitate full recovery:

- Womb experiences that are known or can be found out, where there was violence to the baby or terror, rejection or abuse, or where failed abortion attempts were experienced.
- Possible repressed emotions of terror and overwhelm shown in the child as flickers or meltdowns that seem to come from nowhere and are more dramatic than seen in other children of a similar age.
- Any avoidant or disorganized attachment behaviours where the child doesn't seem bothered by their attachment figure being present or not, or they don't mind which adult they are with.
- Any dissociative behaviour where they may seem to be like different children at different times or they seem to freeze, stare or

zone out for periods of time and seem to lose a sense of being fully alive.

## Children aged 5–9

At this age, children should be full of learning and fascination with the world, with enthusiasm for their hobbies and interests being developed, friends being important and play being central. Puberty is hopefully not quite here yet and so they should be innocent and should be able to play hard and loudly.

These children are still often able to be unashamed about their need for a primary caregiver and can usually snuggle up and enjoy play time and chatting time with them without a sense of shame or embarrassment that they need these adults to help them. If they don't have an emotionally available attachment figure, then they may instead present with anxiety, shame avoidance or fear around adults.

The environment for a child of this age should be one where the child feels that they are welcomed and the behaviour that is appropriate for their age is expected – such as the need to play, experiment, learn and be curious. Anything that is not appropriate for them needs to be carefully hidden or they will undoubtedly find it!

School-age children naturally form habits that may stay with them for life, because what they repeatedly experience becomes 'their normal', especially if the child is able to learn and experiment with things like sweets and unhealthy food. Children of this age are easy to teach, and they learn facts and habits that will impact their whole life. They should also be growing in their ability to use language that has a range of emotional words that they can use to express themselves, and they should be able to express their needs to an adult with a growing degree of confidence.

Children of this age don't often want to talk about their trauma stories if they are asked to, because that sounds too intense and boring. They will, however, usually happily engage with craft, toys and

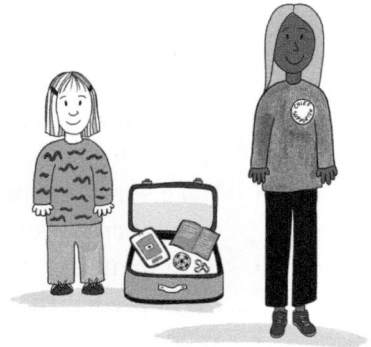

therapeutic games that enable them to express how they feel about life and what has happened. A traumatized child will quickly pick up 'the vibe' of an adult and decide if they like them or not without using many words, but by watching and testing them. It's important to gently make available and facilitate any methods to help support a trauma recovery journey as young as possible, even if they seem to be happy and stable. In this age bracket, it's so much easier to soothe a slight wound that may have occurred in the womb, at birth or in early months of life.

A child this age may demonstrate distress by:

- acting younger than their biological age
- acting more responsibly than is appropriate for their age
- acting aggressively or being stuck in fight or flight mode
- having regular headaches, tummy aches or other physical signs of distress
- wanting to be alone or just wandering around in their 'own world'
- seeming strangely forgetful or seeming to get confused
- having toileting struggles and forgetting or missing the toilet
- not noticing when they are physically hurt and not showing distress at injury
- either being constantly hungry or not being hungry at all
- being easily startled, being jumpy and sensitive to people moving around them
- looking blankly and saying they are fine if anyone asks them
- being sleepy or zoned out
- struggling to engage with learning about things that seem irrelevant to their life
- showing that they are anxious or worried, biting their nails or struggling to sit still
- being angry, sad, tearful or lonely.

Obviously, this list gives a generalized sense of what behaviours and presentations are common following trauma. Every child is unique, but there are some commonalities around children's expression of distress.

## Children aged 10–13

Most of us feel a degree of empathetic pain and we may let out an automatic groan when we think of the time around puberty. It's not an easy time, and adults have to be careful what is said, how we look and how we do most things. As parents, we can quickly embarrass children and can be treated as if we are the most awful thing that they have to admit to having. Children not only desperately need their adult to help guide them through this difficult time but also desperately need to be left alone and given privacy and left to work things out themselves. Getting the right balance is a challenge for most adults who care for these fragile young humans. It is normal for them to push away adults who care for them and sometimes even to reject them with anger, as they battle internally with the feeling of fear of their own vulnerability and powerlessness and the need to feel in control and have power.

These children can sometimes act far younger than they look as if they should, because they may be growing fast physically but, emotionally, they are trying to catch up; or they may act much older than they look as they try and move into being seen as older with less vulnerability and more autonomy.

This age group may be interested in the concept of trauma recovery and so it's important that they are given enough respect for their privacy and for their opinion and thoughts to be heard and valued. They need to feel understood because they often feel scared about how they are being viewed and seen, and so they can look to us as the adults for reassurance. They may hate something that they then love within a minute. They may express strong passions about a topic that they fully deny a day later. This volatility comes with the age and is not necessarily a symptom of distress.

Some children find puberty a time of trauma if it is not carefully and sensitively handled. This age group need their adults to be firm and confident yet relaxed and calm, fun but not stupid, and helpful but not condescending!

So the same therapeutic methods can be used for all ages 5–14 without much adjustment, apart from the way we approach the activities and the 'vibe' we carry, alongside the manner we have as we talk and listen. We must learn quickly when our jokes or language are not what the child deems 'okay' and adjust fast so we don't distract them from the important work of building relationship with us. They need us but they need us to be authentic and genuine, and then they will begin to be curious about us to make sure we really care.

## Children aged 14–18

Teenagers who are mostly through puberty are now slightly less sensitive in some ways but they are still sensitive in other ways. They need the adults around them to keep being attuned enough to recognize when they feel young and small and when they would be horrified to think that we would even know that they sometimes feel like that! They need time and space to explore their identity, their opinions and their thoughts, and they hate to be controlled or ignored.

This means that when we are supporting them through a trauma recovery journey, we need to be able to quickly shift our language and our level of emotional connection to meet their needs so that we are not too intense but at the same time don't seem uncaring or too relaxed about something important.

We need to realize how fast a teenager can sigh and walk away, deciding to wait until we are in a 'better space', when we have no idea what we did! We need to make sure our tone of voice, body posture, facial reactions and language are adjusted appropriately for whatever mood they may be expressing so that we can be the helpful adult that they need us to be. We also need to be relaxed and fast to forgive them when they are rude or unkind to us, and we need to remind ourselves that they just didn't know how to best express their pain.

## Conclusion

This is a very speedy overview of the age differentiations that are essential to understand if we are the adults helping these children navigate their way through to trauma recovery. Most of the activities, methods and ways to facilitate trauma recovery are the same regardless of age, but we need to understand how to 'package' them in the most age-appropriate way, most suited to the specific setting, context and history of each individual child.

THE TRAUMA RECOVERY HANDBOOK

## Questions to reflect on
### For parents/carers/therapeutic mentors

- What words best describe the normal challenges for the age of the child you are thinking about?
- What do you have to be careful to do or not do to help support this child?
- What kind of words or things do they sometimes do that immediately cause you stress and how can you react in a way that is not detrimental to the supportive role you have?
- Have you ever written a basic treatment plan with the main areas that you would like to see restored in the child's life?

### For therapists

- What psychoeducation tools do you use and how have you noticed a reduction in shame?
- Whose treatment plan model are you using? Is it recovery focused and is that clear to all who read it?
- What age do you feel the most relaxed working with and why?
- How do you feel when a child is rude to you or teases you purposely to get a reaction? How do you recover and be able to respond with curiosity?

# CHAPTER 9

# Looking After Yourselves

The fact that you are reading this book shows that you are deeply committed to seeing someone who you care about recovering from what has happened to them. If the child you are supporting has experienced a trauma and you can see the impact in their behaviour or emotions, then you may be reading this hoping you can navigate through to recovery on your own. I hope this book does help you feel more confident and calmer as you decide to do all you can for that child.

It is recognized by those of us who work in this field that it can be exhausting for the adult who is the primary caregiver to the struggling child. In aeroplanes, when the announcement comes to make sure that adults put their oxygen masks on before helping the children near them put theirs on, I do reflect on how hard that would be in a crisis. It can be instinctive to first give up our own freedom, time and energy to help those more vulnerable than ourselves. It can also be a driving motivator that we want to help these children navigate their journey with maybe more ease than we had, and certainly with more support and kindness to cheer them on. Bessel van der Kolk (2014) explains that 'trauma affects not only those who are directly exposed to it, but also those around them' (p.1).

For example, what do we do when a child:

- refuses to do anything we suggest
- refuses to come off screens/go to therapy/move
- is stuck in fight mode and seems to just fight everyone?

The problem is that there is no miracle answer that would be fully applicable to the exhaustion or stress that you may be feeling because each child is different, but the reason the child is behaving like this is due to them trying to cope with their own inner turmoil. It's not easy, it's not simple, and it can be exhausting trying to help those who ask for help in the most painful ways. We also recognize that they can take a long time to learn to trust us and that trust has to be tested, again and again.

## Secondary stress and the trauma of building relationships with traumatized children

What we do know is that spending time with children who are volatile, angry, frustrated, emotionally dysregulated and irritable can be extremely exhausting and can sometimes feel like an impossible task. You may have been kicked, spat at, shouted at, screamed at, told that it is all your fault and lied to, and felt that you didn't even have the energy to defend yourself. In those moments, it can feel deeply unfair, utterly painful and as if your life is hopeless and beyond help. You may feel that people have no idea of what you live with (and they probably don't understand how relentless it may be or feel), and they may offer you simple answers that can make you want to scream further or say with a degree of absolute horror, 'Don't you think I may have thought of that?' It can feel endless, agony, beyond exhausting and relentless. Ironically, it can be possible that you develop trauma symptoms because you are helping the child with their trauma symptoms – and yet the biggest stress often comes from those offering you their opinion or assumptions without authentic empathy, care and genuine support.

Brené Brown (2021) describes the impact of stressful situations. She says that they can:

> cause both physiological (body) and psychological (mind and emotion) reactions. However, regardless of how strongly our body responds to stress (increases in heart rate and cortisol), our emotional reaction is more tied to our cognitive assessment of whether we can cope with the situation than to how our body is coping. (p.6)

This helps us understand that our body is responding to our thoughts rather than warning us that we aren't coping. This is hopeful because we can focus on 'catching' those negative thought spirals where things can begin to feel hopeless and then concentrate on a few themes in our mind, such as knowing that others have managed to walk this path to better days, we are not alone and this is worth our investment, time and sacrifice. These positive affirmations can begin to help us find enough hope to keep going when we feel it is too much.

## Looking for the glimmers

Within the stress of the role of supporter, it is easy to see the things that are going wrong, but it is vital to also see the tiny signs of growth and change. Just like a seed that is planted and watered, it can feel hopeless until you see the tiniest sprout of life. The tiny signs of life with traumatized children can go unnoticed unless you choose to look for them and celebrate them. Some of us call them glimmers that can be found, like a shiny shell on a beach full of stones, while triggers are the large, very visible rocks that sometimes trip the child up or cause them to wobble, stumble or scream. To be emotionally available for the traumatized child through the long journey of recovery, it is vital that every adult feels able to do some things which may feel selfish but are life giving and essential for them to endure the long run until there is stability and health.

## Your own trauma recovery journey as an adult

It's also important to remember that no matter how we feel as we start this intentional journey of support, we, as normal humans, may find some aspects of it tough and challenging. It may bring up some of our own wounds, disappointments, traumatic experiences and frustrations. We need to recognize that when this happens, it is not because we are failing, or we are now unhelpful. If it is at all possible, while you work hard to help the child recover from trauma, take some time to then treat yourself in the same way. I would suggest making a list of what to do when you feel overwhelmed or exhausted.

- Who can you be honest with – on the phone, text or over a coffee?
- What brings comfort to you that you can make sure you give yourself regularly?

127

- Are you able to eat well and exercise?
- How do you unwind when you feel full of unexpressed anxiety or frustration?
- Who are your support team?
- What would you say to a friend going through the same thing?

Ideally, all adults who are in the position of primary cheerleader, nurturer, co-regulator and comforter would benefit from some kind of group where they can talk, listen, find support and share ideas, preferably with a facilitator who is trained to offer suggestions with no shame or judgement but rather empathy and kindness. If possible, therapy that can offer similar qualities of not judging, fixing or shaming, and kind, gentle and affirming support can provide personal space where you can feel supported and can process the challenges.

When you are the adult caring for a child, it can be surprising to find childhood traumatic experiences that you had maybe thought had been forgotten or 'dealt with' resurfacing. Sometimes the adult can find themselves grieving over things that did or didn't happen to them as a child, or remembering small or larger traumatic experiences that seem to have risen from the depth of their unconscious or subconscious. This is very common, and there doesn't need to be any panic or shame about it as we are all humans with a history of being around other humans where difficult things can happen. One of our clever coping mechanisms to help us survive is to bury memories away from our everyday life so that we can continue to live day to day and achieve what we want to. A lot of adults find that when they are caring for children, they suddenly remember things that happened to them when they were the age of the child whom they are caring for.

It is important to find some help so that you can navigate the complexities of caring for a child with trauma and your own childhood memories resurfacing, because things can go a little bit wrong when the two become muddled in a tired and overwhelmed brain. It is important to have someone who can remind you of some elements of your story and keep that separate from the child's story and memories. These people can be a bit like the guardrail or bumpers on a bowling alley, which stop the heavy balls that are thrown going into the wrong lanes or knocking into other people's bowling balls.

## Intergenerational trauma recovery

Some of you reading this book may be aware that the children you are supporting are living through similar experiences to those you went through as a child. It's possible that you are aware that there has been a generational pattern of abuse, neglect or relational trauma and so you may feel more frustrated or angry or more accepting of what has happened. It can be possible to view this journey as a challenge but also a privilege to help a child recover from trauma and know that as they journey towards recovery, they will have skills and knowledge that will enable them to heal the generational pattern and create a hope-filled future where they are ready to help others understand some aspects of their own needs and rights as children. Well done to you if you are on this journey and you are focused on not just seeing recovery for one child but also their children!

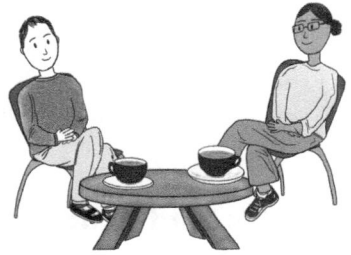

## Your inner child

As an adult, you may find the concept of having an inner child bizarre, but it is possible that there is a part of you that misses being young or feels a little bit stuck in being sad about the things that happened when you were little. It could be that part of you is still looking to be rescued or supported from when you were a child, and no one seemed to appear. This could be an indicator that your inner child needs some time from you, to be heard and validated. You can just take a few minutes a day, maybe in the car on your own after a school drop-off, or in the evening you can have a five-minute walk around the block where you can speak with that younger part of you and reassure them that you care, that you know it is unfair that you didn't have that support when you were little, but that you are trying now to listen and care for them. It may sound weird, but you may find that you can spend a little longer allowing the odd memory to resurface and validating it, maybe feeling some of the feelings that got stuck and acknowledging the injustice of the situation. This can decrease some internal stress and turmoil and enable you to continue to take the role of chief supporter for the children in your world with less dis-ease.

'If I am honest, I think I was angry that he had more love and things than I ever had but he was still angry at me. So, we often got caught in a cycle of both being angry at each other. Actually, we were just both sad and needed to be honest. Then I could be the dad he needed.' *Father of son aged 13*

## It is hard to do it alone

If you are the supporter for a child who needs the safety and stability of your relationship while you are also needing to recover from the trauma from your childhood, life or from the experience of helping this child, and so you have been the main focus of their emotional dysregulation, you may feel as if all the plates are in the air and something could drop at any point. It is important to remember a few things at this point:

- You are doing the best you can.
- Things won't be like this forever.
- You are important too and you have needs that are okay to acknowledge.
- Anyone who judges you doesn't know your whole story, so ignore them.
- Lots of people are stressed, so try hard not to take whatever is said to you personally.
- Someone may have something helpful to say amid the misunderstanding, so don't ignore it all! Wisdom can come from funny places!

At the core of an understanding of trauma recovery is the recognition that we need others in our lives to be able to live well. It can be that there is a support group in your area, or you could maybe try and start one. This would purely be a space for adults to be able to share news in a supportive environment with people who won't judge, shame, gossip or mock anything that another brings to the space, but are able to listen carefully, empathize, be there emotionally to offer tissues and coffee and jointly create an emotionally safe space to support each other. It is important that you have a space where you can explore and reflect on your own nervous system, how you are feeling and what you could do to get stronger and more able to keep being the place of safety for others.

## It's worth the effort and time

It really is worth the continual effort to be emotionally available, smile when you see them, give them more than you feel you have at the time and co-regulate with them, even when you may want to scream or run away. The dilemma is that if you feel as if you can't do it anymore, then your attention and emotional availability will be inconsistent and so the child may become more demanding and the other trauma symptoms may escalate further. Gabor Maté (1999) explains this beautifully:

> Understandably the parent may long for respite, not more engagement. The conundrum is that attention given at the request of the child is never satisfactory; it leaves an uncertainty that the parent is only responding to demands, not voluntarily giving of himself, of herself, to the child. The demands only escalate, without the emotional need underlying them ever being filled. The solution is to seize the moment, to invite contact exactly when the child is not demanding it. (p.154)

## Conclusion

The role of carer for a traumatized child can be difficult and overwhelming, but when we are able to be honest enough to admit that we do sometimes all make mistakes, we are not perfect, we can have bad days, we can crave personal space some days and caring can feel relentless, it can feel less painful. Obviously, no adult can be perfect, strong all the time or have all the knowledge that they need, but we can decide to laugh at the disasters (in a way that doesn't cause shame for the child) and keep a sense of humour on the journey.

Ultimately, it is vital for all adults to be a part of a larger group who choose to intentionally journey in understanding trauma recovery, so that there is less isolation and an increased sense of support. Parental support and empowerment are a key element of the Trauma Recovery Focused Model®.

## Questions to reflect on
### For parents/carers/therapeutic mentors

- Who have you got in your world who you can debrief with or find support?
- Have you experienced childhood trauma that is now beginning to be apparent and so you may need some therapy?
- What things can you do for yourself that make you feel more human and less exhausted?
- What things that the child does are specific triggers for you and how can you prepare to be less reactive?
- What do you find the hardest thing to do as an adult who is supporting a traumatized child and what can you do to help make it less difficult?
- What can you look forward to?
- What activity can you do with the child that both you and they enjoy?

### For therapists

- How are you supporting the parent/carer with information and ideas to help them?
- What practices do you use to help yourself with the stress and secondary trauma of the work and how are you planning to do this long term?

# THE GENERAL AREAS OF IMPACT

CHAPTER 10

# Shame, Post-Traumatic Growth and Other Vital Elements

This book is aimed at helping you the adult enable a child or young person to navigate through to trauma recovery. The first section explores the vital foundations that need to be built to enable the healing and recovery to take place. When a child is able to begin to feel safe emotionally and environmentally, and have positive therapeutic supportive relationships in place, then they can begin the journey of recovering from the awful experiences that they endured. Without the content of Section 1 being applied, any healing or recovery will be like a house built on mud – it won't last a long time and will eventually collapse! It sadly just can't be rushed, unless the child has experienced a Type I single-incident trauma, in which case it can sometimes be fast to recover, especially if the child already has some positive relationships which can be supportive and intentional to help facilitate recovery.

I do recognize how frustrating that is, especially if you are navigating your way through a traumatic journey yourself and you are trying to offer a safe environment and relationship, but you are living immersed in your own trauma. In this situation, you need to draw on any other positive, consistent relationships that you can find to strengthen the safety for your child – friends, relatives and professionals who will commit to longer-term support.

If you are a professional who is limited to short-term work or who has to primarily focus on the delivery of curriculum or other specific outcomes that are measured, I recognize the limitation of your time and the boundaries of your role, and the frustration that you may be the only adult in the life of the child who holds hope for them to recover. Your belief in them, your relationship with them that provides some emotional safety and hope, can be life changing for them, so I would suggest that you explore the elements of recovery in this book and then facilitate what you can do within the time that you have, with careful reflection on how to avoid any experiences where they are brave enough to be vulnerable and then they feel ignored, misunderstood or rushed on to another issue that needs to be considered. If they experience a positive relationship with you, where they can sense that you believe that they have hope and a future, then that will probably stay with them for their whole life – so well done.

## Shame – the invisible thread of destruction

Shame is present when trauma has happened, like an invisible defender that is also a silent destroyer. When a child experiences trauma, due to the appropriately egotistical nature of a child which enables them to survive, they assume subconsciously that what happened to them was their fault. This may make no sense to us, but it is the nature of childhood and how children perceive the world. Perpetrators know this and assume that even when they inflict the worst trauma on a child, the child will probably not disclose for a long time, possibly decades, because they will assume it was their fault.

I have written a whole book about shame, *The Simple Guide to Understanding Shame in Children*, because of the centrality of it to trauma recovery and again I cannot repeat it here because it is 30,000 words in length! But it is essential reading and here is a snippet:

> When shame is experienced, it functions as an urgent signal that danger is here: the danger of rejection, failure, exposure and abandonment. It is an experience rooted in interpersonal relationships. It threatens the very basic human experience of being alive and needing to belong, be loved and be accepted.
>
> We know that the experience of shame induces a sudden sense of fear that is instinctive and not a considered reaction. This instinctive fear seems to be coupled with a sense of panic, which is a reaction more suited to obvious danger or threat.

If a child experiences shame occasionally, they are able to recover and move on and it doesn't necessarily have a negative impact, but if they are exposed to regular experiences of shame, they can develop negative coping mechanisms which can cause significant toxic stress and have a lasting impact on their relationships, emotions, behaviour and learning. Coping mechanisms will be explored in the following chapters but could include lying, pretending, avoiding challenging situations, running away or hating themselves.

## The difference between shame and guilt

Shame is different from guilt because shame is usually interpreted as 'I am bad and you think I am bad' whereas guilt is interpreted as 'I did something bad'. This thought process takes place at a subconscious level, meaning it happens internally so the person is not aware of these feelings and beliefs, although they do affect their behaviour. Guilt means that the child can usually 'fix' the problem by apologizing for the bad thing they did. However, when a child feels that they themselves are bad and believes that people around them think they are too, they can feel that they are not loved and wanted because they are bad and so a feeling of rejection can begin to form. This feeling can cause terror as they simultaneously subconsciously realize that they are reliant on adults to meet their needs and rejection therefore feels like a life or death issue.

Another way of putting it would be that guilt says you made a mistake but shame says that you are a mistake. Many traumatized children live with a core sense of being a mistake and sadly continue to live lives trying to soothe the painful, deep feelings of fundamentally being a mistake and worthless.

Contrastingly, guilt can be a helpful experience that can lead to improved interpersonal skills if the person experiencing it is able to do something about the uncomfortable feeling. For example, if a child hits their friend because they want a toy and then that friend cries, it can be helpful to be able to help the child to pause and notice the crying child and point out their reaction to being hit. This can lead to guilt which can motivate the child to ask to borrow the toy in future. (de Thierry, 2018, pp.16–17)

## The Shame Continuum

We need to grasp the difference between the different levels of shame that exist in humans and so the Shame Continuum (diagram below) was created to help explore the different levels and what that impact could be in someone's life.

There is the kind of shame that we all experience when we feel stupid or embarrassed and we feel the gaze of others in our moment of stupidity, compared to the shame that is experienced due to a situation of abuse or a horrid secret that an adult makes a child carry. This compares to the most extreme end of shame where a person feels that they themselves are faulty, and although this belief sits at a subconscious or unconscious level, the person's behaviour and thinking are based on this core belief. This is often due to developmental trauma.

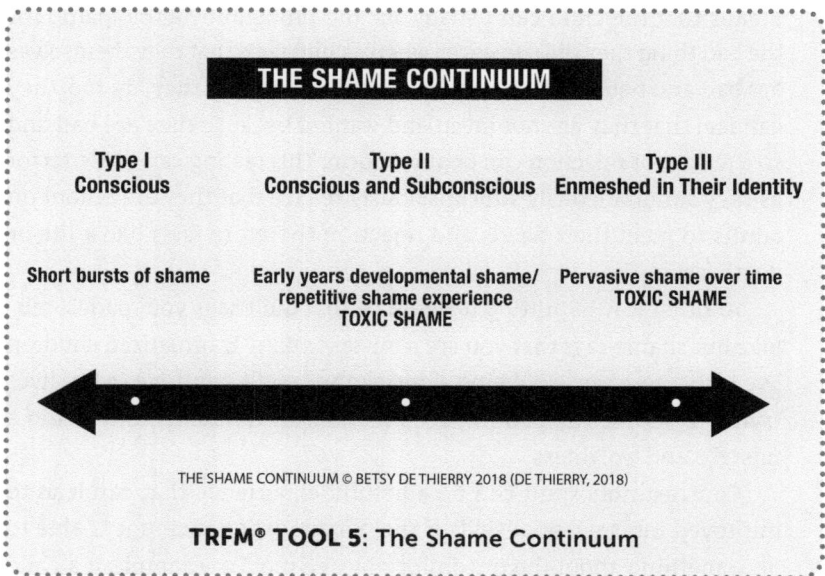

### THE SHAME CONTINUUM

| Type I | Type II | Type III |
|---|---|---|
| Conscious | Conscious and Subconscious | Enmeshed in Their Identity |
| Short bursts of shame | Early years developmental shame/ repetitive shame experience TOXIC SHAME | Pervasive shame over time TOXIC SHAME |

THE SHAME CONTINUUM © BETSY DE THIERRY 2018 (DE THIERRY, 2018)

**TRFM® TOOL 5:** The Shame Continuum

Without being in any way able to summarize the book, which explores every symptom and behaviour that is rooted in shame and what to do to reduce it, here is a little summary of what the impact is and what we need to do to reduce the shame.

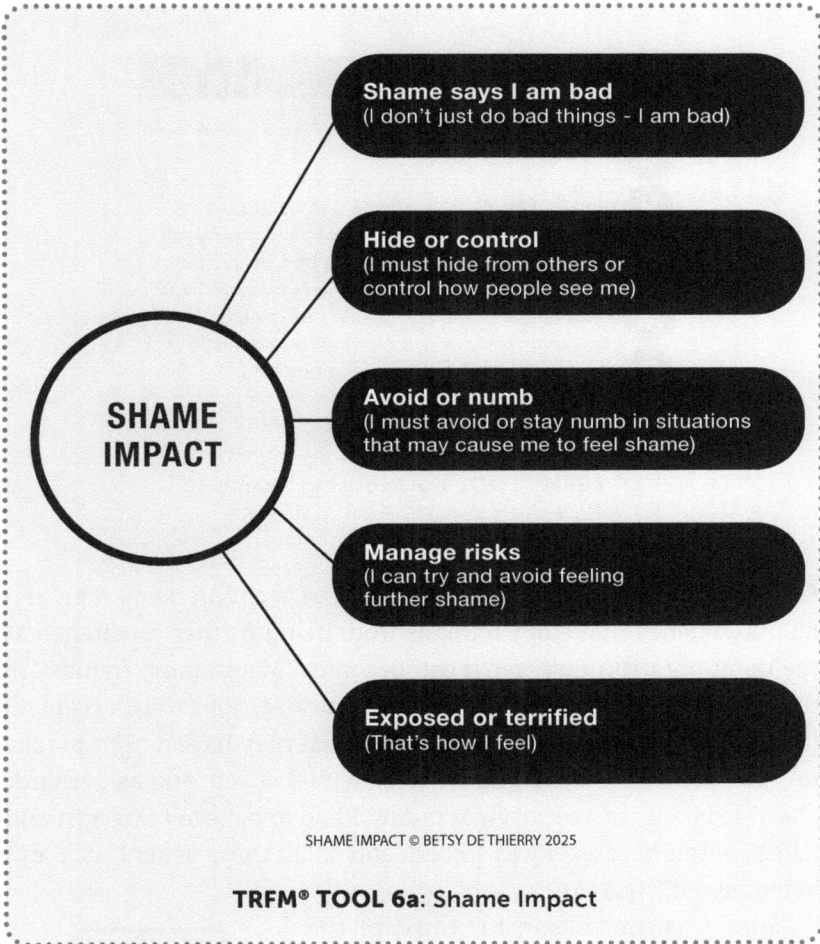

**SHAME IMPACT**

**Shame says I am bad**
(I don't just do bad things - I am bad)

**Hide or control**
(I must hide from others or control how people see me)

**Avoid or numb**
(I must avoid or stay numb in situations that may cause me to feel shame)

**Manage risks**
(I can try and avoid feeling further shame)

**Exposed or terrified**
(That's how I feel)

SHAME IMPACT © BETSY DE THIERRY 2025

**TRFM® TOOL 6a**: Shame Impact

## SHAME impact

The person who feels shame ends up avoiding being further exposed and rejected and lives in terror of that happening. This causes them to build a lot of different defences to enable them to survive the feelings of terror of what could happen. To recover from shame, several elements are needed, including recognition of the impact of it, the reason for it and the most common coping strategies that could be used.

## SHAME

**S**hame is not guilt

**H**abits that come from shame can be hidden

**A**cknowledging that others have hurt us is vital

**M**oving out of hiding and taking risk is hard

**E**xposing the lies of shame is important

EXPOSING SHAME © BETSY DE THIERRY 2025

**TRFM® TOOL 6b: Exposing Shame**

Shame needs to be exposed and explored with children and seen as a helpful defence that stops humans from being further threatened at the point of terror; however, it can become a life-draining framework through which the child has to fight to survive, fight to be accepted, fight to not be rejected and fight to feel that they have a right to take up space. Shame and trauma are deeply interwoven, and as Gerhardt (2004) explains, 'as one survivor put it, "I had to believe I was hurt and hated myself because I was so bad, and so all these years I hurt and hated myself"' (p.143).

Shame is the reason for most of the challenging behaviours that make children look as if they are defiant, they don't care, they want power, or they withdraw or hide or hate themselves. It is vital that shame is explored at length, to be able to reduce its power and help the child feel the weight taken off them. They need to know that it was never their fault and what happened to them was unfair and unjust and they are *not* bad people, but people who have been hurt and need care.

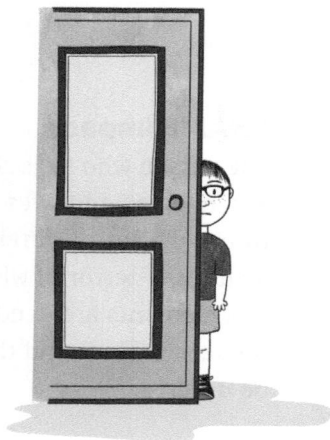

'I think I had given up on myself because I kept getting into trouble. I didn't know why and my head was spinning because I was trying hard but I just got into fights and stuff. I wanted to be good and then hated myself and thought I'd be like this forever. Now I get it more. That I am scared and need to go to a safe space to calm down. Sometimes I even cry now. That's because Miss S helps me know I'm not bad, I'm sad.' *Sam, aged 9*

## Vulnerability

Trauma recovery takes courage. It is courageous to acknowledge that we were hurt and that injustice occurred. It is courageous to speak about it even once, let alone go on a journey of acknowledging that not only did it happen but it also impacted many areas of our lives. It takes courage to feel feelings that were too much to feel at the time of the pain, and then reflect on them and acknowledge their purpose. It takes courage to recognize the defence mechanism and coping mechanisms that have become so familiar but were never meant to be adopted as normal. It takes courage to know that some children live carefree, happy, innocent and protected lives, are loved and celebrated and know none of the turmoil, pain, confusion, overwhelm and powerlessness of trauma.

Having the courage to be vulnerable and not stay in the armour of using defence mechanisms that guard against the fear of anyone seeing that vulnerability and therefore being able to abuse us further can be terrifying. Vulnerability is not easy, it is not cost free, and it is a risk. Anyone working with traumatized children or adults must realize that the very nature of being traumatized means that their trust in adults has been broken, causing significant damage. Vulnerability is needed for the journey of recovery – through every moment of realization, every moment of needing to choose courage, to remember, admit and acknowledge that the feelings that come feel life altering, life defining, exhausting and far 'too much' for any human to own and carry. Brené Brown (2021) says that 'vulnerability is not weakness; it's our greatest measure of courage' (p.14).

When we are able to support someone who is on this journey of trauma recovery, we need to be aware of what it costs for them to walk through it, how often the emotions feel too much and the body groans and feels exhausted and wrung dry, while only small steps seem to be made. They may feel as if they are beginning to look weak and could be perceived as being weak, but we need to make sure that they realize we are aware of how courageous they are being to not deny the reality of the pain.

> To emotionally connect with others takes vulnerability, and even to love another involves the risk of being rejected, yet it is a core aspect of becoming and being healthy. When people have been hurt in a relationship, they need to heal in a relationship. We need to be 'vulnerability detectors' though, so that we detect quickly when a child or adult is being vulnerable with us and react with appropriate empathy and kindness. What could be normal chat to us could be courageous vulnerability for them. For some people who are testing out being vulnerable, these early attempts at sharing their thoughts or feelings can lead either to trust being built or to further withdrawal if their attempts are met with insensitivity. (de Thierry, 2019, pp.95–96)

Vulnerability is essential on the journey, but it needs to be honoured and never expected. It should be respected and acknowledged and never misused or abused or treated as casual.

## The ongoing trauma journey and post-traumatic growth

We must hold the tension that while the trauma recovery journey can sometimes feel never-ending, there is a sense of it being possible for the child to fully move on. However, it is important to note that at any period of life when there is a new stressor, such as puberty, a change of school, exams, a new relationship, a relationship breakdown or a new or different job, there may well be a return of some old trauma coping mechanism that was unresolved. This doesn't mean that the child is 'back to where they started' and so 'what was the point of those years of working hard on their emotional health'; because it is usually just a wobble or a blip. It is in these short moments that the child or young person needs supportive adults to remind them of how far they have come and how much life they have lived without any interruption from the trauma symptoms. They can usually soon regain their confidence and be able to move forward.

Post-traumatic growth is also a reality that must not be overlooked! This is a concept that is important to recognize, because when a child has been through this trauma recovery process over many years, they often become more self-aware and more relationally and emotionally intelligent than some of their peers. It's a little bit like the broken leg that is now stronger than before the break because it has been in a plaster cast and rested and the child has had to focus on lots of specific exercises to develop strength.

> Psychologists Richard Tedeschi, PhD and Lawrence Calhoun, PhD (2004) wrote about the way that sometimes humans can actually also experience positive elements to the recovery of their trauma, which can be referred to as post-traumatic growth. This does not deny the pain and turmoil of the traumatic experiences, but merely shows that there is research that has found that growth often co-exists with the continuing distress of the trauma. They discovered that, following a traumatic experience, children and young people can often feel more compassion and empathy for others, a deeper understanding of personal values, purpose and meaning in life; they can also place a greater value on interpersonal relationships. Also, they were found to have increased psychological and emotional maturity and a more 'complex appreciation of life' compared to others of a similar age. (de Thierry, 2021, p.98)

The rest of Section 2 will explore the different areas that may be impacted by the traumatic experience. It may be obvious as you look at the title of a chapter that the child you are caring for has been impacted in that way, but it may also be that the impact is more hidden.

## Our own stories

Many of us who understand trauma have had personal experiences of trauma and my life is no exception. Our stories hold the hope that it's possible to survive and then process and recover from what has happened. We all have stories to tell and often those with a deep intuitive understanding of trauma have chosen to find ways to describe our experiences in a way that would bring understanding to many more people about the terror, powerlessness and overwhelm that is felt so deeply. Our stories need to be told, and we all need to continue to lean in and listen to others so that we can deepen our understanding of the painful impact of trauma, so that we can continue to bring support and champion others on the road to recovery.

It's been my privilege to hear many stories from the many thousands of children, young people and adults that I have supported through a trauma recovery journey. It's also been a privilege to train other professionals to hold the knowledge that trauma recovery is possible. This recovery journey has been evidenced through data from the charity I founded, The Trauma Recovery Centre, which has been professionally evaluated by Christ Church Canterbury University to show that 98.8% of children have made significant progress.

So, I am cheering you on in your own journey and that of all those children and families who you work with. I believe that our mess can become our message, our stories can bring hope for others and post-traumatic growth is a reality!

I wholeheartedly agree with Brené Brown when she says that:

> The opposite of recognizing that we're feeling something is denying our emotions. The opposite of being curious is disengaging. When we deny our stories and disengage from tough emotions, they don't go away; instead, they own us, they define us. Our job is not to deny the story, but to defy the ending – to rise strong, recognize our story, and rumble with the truth until we get to a place where we think, Yes. This is what happened. This is my truth. And I will choose how this story ends. (Brown, 2015, p.50)

## General areas that are impacted by trauma

- The body and nervous system.
- The emotions and regulation.
- The mind.
- The subconscious and unconscious.
- Their relationships.

The following chapters will explore where the trauma impacts these different areas and when it is time to ask for help because the symptoms seem to be getting worse and so the child needs more help. It's important to recognize that some trauma experiences seem to generate more empathy and kindness when their stories are told than others. When some trauma experiences are shared, the listener can seem to minimize the reality of the level of courage it took the person to share their story and they may shrug their shoulders or compare with someone else's story or look uninterested. This can be deeply distressing and can cause the person to not share their painful story again. Others seem to react with fear or disgust at some stories and can then seem to behave differently towards the person who shared. That is horrific and retraumatizing to the person who has hoped that sharing their story may begin to bring strength for their recovery.

Often, single-incident traumatic experiences evoke more empathy because people can identify with the horror of a car crash or the death of a loved one, while emotional or financial abuse or neglect can often be over-simplified and ignored. Emotional neglect is also often brushed aside despite research that it is more damaging than many other abuses.

## How does trauma recovery happen?

These are the TRFM® signs we look for as the foundations of being ready for further trauma recovery work. The foundations are usually facilitated by parents, carers and therapeutic mentors.

### Foundations of understanding trauma

- The adults understand trauma and what the impact is. Then there is less likelihood that they will misunderstand the behaviour and emotions of the child and make wrong assumptions.
- The adults are able to reflect on the trauma continuum and if the child is Type I, II or III, and therefore they can differentiate between 'normal' childhood behaviour and behaviour that indicates distress.

### Foundations of relationships

- The adults can understand the role of relationships in the recovery from trauma. They can explore and grow confident in key skills such as emotional connection through attunement, validation, non-verbal communication and spending time doing things that are enjoyable for the child to do with the adult.

- The child can identify the key adults who are building the attachment relationship with them.

## Foundations for safe environments

- The adults can understand and reflect on the environments that the child spends time in. How are they conducive to feeling safe and healing? Is there anything the adult could do to change them or make them feel safer.
- The school is aware of any of the triggers for the child and has a plan for when they need a safe place.

## Foundation of the bigger picture

- Healthy habits begin to be seen as part of a healthy foundation.
- A method has been chosen to track the child's ups and downs so that progress can be seen over time.

## Foundation for the supporting adults

- Some support can be thought through for the adults who are facilitating safety and recovery. How are the adults supporting themselves? What could they do to increase this?
- The adults and children grow in being able to communicate key elements of psychoeducation.

This is a brief overview and is discussed further in Chapter 26.

## Conclusion

Understanding the power of shame can transform all our lives if we are able to reflect on our vulnerability as a human who is built to need community and belonging. Children need to know that we care for them and understand that their behaviour is communication and they are on a journey to recovery and growth. There should be no shame in our stories of trauma, and post-traumatic growth is possible!

This section of the book has explored the areas of a child's life that need to be reflected on so that they can experience a growing sense of safety and stability. With the foundations of long-term positive nurturing relationships, environmental and emotional safety, healthy habits and the knowledge that those adults who are surrounding them understand what trauma symptoms are, children are able to take positive steps towards healing. These aspects of a child's life act like the foundations of a house, enabling the child to courageously explore the deeper and more specific trauma impact that is the focus of the following section. While this list of areas that need to be explored looks like a tick sheet, the reality is that we as humans are complex and the child may some days seem to be making significant progress and then other days may seem to struggle – but the wiggly path to recovery still starts with these solid and vital foundations. Well done to all of you for supporting, building, helping and being emotionally present for these children who need you.

## Questions to reflect on
### For parents/carers/therapeutic mentors

- Where do you think the child is 'up to' on the list of areas to be worked on?
- What shame symptoms have you noticed in the child?
- What ways have you found to reduce the shame they feel?
- Do they struggle with vulnerability?
- Can you see any signs of post-traumatic growth? Or how can you remember to hold on to that as hope for the future?

### For therapists

- How do you monitor shame in the child's relationships?
- How do you intentionally reduce shame when trauma is the focus?
- How do you help the child feel safe when they are being vulnerable?

# CHAPTER 11

# The Impact of Trauma on the Body

## The automatic survival reaction

When humans suddenly feel frightened, we have automatic, instinctive reactions that are designed to save our lives. The 'fight or flight response' was a term first used by US physiologist Walter Cannon (1871–1945) to describe the physiological responses of being confronted with a situation that evokes fear, pain or anger. He described the fast, unconscious and automatic reactions that occur inside the body to survive a threat.

The concept has been developed further over the decades to understand the possibility of other more adaptive responses:

- Fight: either physically or with defensive words.
- Flight: we run away or go into denial.
- Freeze: we literally become motionless, or we dissociate.
- Flop: we either fall to the floor or become exhausted or stuck.
- Fawn: we develop people-pleasing reactions to avoid conflict.

Although these mechanisms are clever, vital and possibly did save our lives in the instant of the first traumatic experience, they sadly become the automatic mechanism that reacts to any terror or powerlessness in the same way. There are further consequences because:

the immediate release of adrenalin (epinephrine) that prepares the person to fight or to flee then leads to increased blood pressure, accelerated heart rate, increased sweating, dilation of the pupils, diversion of blood flow from the digestive tract to the skeletal muscles and cessation of digestive processes, release of sugar from reserves in the liver and other symptoms. (Colman, 2008, p.162)

When we are afraid, our thinking brain cannot process the difference between an actual threat and something that could be a threat, and so our nervous system reacts as if it is life threatening. That's why sometimes children and adults who have experienced trauma have what could be called exaggerated, extreme and abnormal reactions to a small situation. Our brains and nervous system can't work out how probable the threat is without the use of our cognitive reasoning. When we become more aware of the instinctive reaction to anything that reminds us of threat, then we cannot overrule it cognitively and it becomes our natural reaction to even the tiniest bit of threat.

## The impact of shock and terror

This immediate impact on the body of a threat and trauma is usually experienced as a big shock – whether it was a physical shock like being hit on the head or pushed to the ground or an emotional shock such as a terrifying scream or sight, it becomes stored in our memory bank as something that needs to be defended against. This means that anything in life that seems to hold the possibility of retraumatization can cause the past unprocessed experiences to unconsciously instruct the body to react again as if the person were in danger. Shell shock was first mentioned in medical literature in 1915 by Myers in a study of veterans.

It can be really embarrassing for children and young people, and friends may laugh or tease them for having such a wildly inappropriate reaction to something small. Many traumatized children know the pain of these reactions from others, and sadly, as adults, we recognize that they are usually quite innocent comments that are due to a lack of understanding of the impact of trauma.

This is why some children and young people have made sure they look as if they don't care. They have decided that if they do let anyone know they care, they may have to experience the devastation of people not responding in the way they need them to, so it's easier to pretend it doesn't matter anyway. Some children may smile or laugh all the time and even be known for being cheery, but it is often a coping mechanism so that people don't question what is going on in their lives and come too close. The smile keeps people at a distance so that their frightening secrets will remain untold and further punishment for telling anyone what went on won't happen.

Van der Kolk (2014) explains how the body holds the pain of the past:

> What has happened cannot be undone. But what can be dealt with are the imprints of the trauma on body, mind and soul; the crushing sensations in your chest that you may label as anxiety or depression; the fear of losing control; always being on alert for danger or rejection; the self-loathing; the nightmares and flashbacks; the fog that keeps you from staying on task and from engaging fully in what you are doing; being unable to fully open up your heart to another human being. Trauma robs you of the feeling that you are in charge of yourself. Of what I call self-leadership in the chapters to come. The challenge of recovery is to re-establish ownership of your body and your mind – of yourself. This means feeling free to know what you know and to feel what you feel without becoming overwhelmed, enraged, ashamed or collapsed. (p.205)

## Body pain

Our bodies send messages to our brains all day long, whether it is to remind ourselves to eat and drink or to use the toilet. We can feel it in our chest when we must take an uncomfortable phone call and we can feel twitchy and restless when we need to walk outside or get some exercise. Children should develop an understanding of what their body is trying to communicate with these signs, but often when they have been experiencing trauma, they are disconnected from these feelings due to their overwhelm and coping mechanisms that stop them feeling, like dissociation. For many children, there are just too many body messages, and they would love it to be as simple as food, drink, toilet and exercise, with the odd feeling of glee and joy thrown in. Instead, these vulnerable children have to process the normal feelings of being alive alongside many other signs and signals of distress and discomfort, both emotionally and physically. Children with developmental trauma frequently experience chronic abdominal pain, headaches, chest pain, fainting and seizure-like episodes – all very common symptoms related to a sensitized stress response (Perry & Winfrey, 2022, p.141).

If a child is living through terror and powerlessness, the impact of the experience can sit inside their tummies like a massive knot that is tied so hard it stops them breathing.

They may feel that their legs have no power in them, and when the teacher says to walk to another room, they can't feel them and wonder what to do.

They may have a burning sensation in their private parts due to abuse that is now a body memory, which confuses them because while the abuse has stopped, they wonder why they still feel flashes of pain or as if a fire is between their legs, and they also panic about who else can see.

They may not notice that they haven't needed the toilet for several days or they may dissociate when they go to the toilet because they cannot cope with the body sensations that they feel or the knowledge that those areas of the body even exist.

They may hate exercise because the sensation of their breathing changing and their heart beating can be terrifying and feel as if they are dying.

They may eat the lunch provided at school and then eat anyone else's that they can see because they cannot feel the sensation of being full. They switched off that feeling when their home no longer had enough food for everyone because the feeling of hunger was too painful and interruptive.

They may have endured childhood surgery or long-term frightening health treatment and been totally confused by the adults who seemed to be so kind but who then hurt them and caused them to scream so that 'they would get better'. Now they are not sure they like adults.

Many of these children have had to learn to stop feeling their bodily feelings to keep going through the daily rhythm of life as they are expected to do, but it means that they no longer know easily how to feel their hunger, thirst, pain from a wound, their need to use a toilet or if they feel sick or emotionally distressed. The sensations have been blocked out or numbed.

The body can hold the memories of the trauma. Sometimes the pain that the body can be left with longer term is directly linked, such as pain in the genital area due to abuse, or pain in the chest where the child was crushed. While the child may not remember the details of the experience and so have no memory of the event, the body remembers and the pain remains, usually coming and going inconsistently, as if it is still happening. Very often it's the body that remembers the feelings that came as a result of the traumatic event, such as the struggle to breathe, the tummy ache and sick feelings that they were left with, the headache and dizziness, the fear of the dark, or wrists feeling tender. The child may well speak about these pains because they are often not aware that they are linked to the trauma, but sadly adults can often brush them off as exaggeration or lying because they can't say when the pain started and what happened. The child can also be left hypersensitive to smells, visual stimuli and sounds as they try and avoid anything that reminds their subconscious of the experience. They may become mute or lethargic as physiological and emotional responses to overwhelm. (de Thierry, 2020, pp.33–34)

## How to recover from body pains and notice automatic reactions

The child can recover and learn to be in tune with their body, but the first step is for them to understand how their body works. They need help to understand how we function as humans and how we have automatic reactions that we can teach ourselves to override, but how that is not helpful in the long term.

There are some fantastic therapeutic story books and videos available to help children begin to understand how normal it is to have these reactions. This psychoeducation reduces shame so that they can learn about themselves; otherwise, the shame of feeling weird or different or faulty causes them to be uninterested and to be defensive instead.

When they can understand that brains sometimes misinterpret information, we can then talk them through different scenarios where sometimes a child may have an inappropriate reaction or doesn't notice something that seems obvious to others around them.

The most important thing for the child who may be disconnected from their body or may be experiencing different body pains is to understand how clever their body is to survive frightening things and to begin to want to learn more about how the nervous system works.

Then they need to be able to reflect with an adult on instances where they have seen themselves lose a sense of calm and become hyperaroused or hypoaroused, and what they wish they could have done when they felt those feelings. It could be that they needed to 'discharge the energy' they felt at a time when they were triggered by something, so it can be helpful to create with them a similar but not at all traumatizing story where they feel annoyed or angry, and for them to run or fight or flop as they would have wanted to but weren't able to. They may also then need to process the memory of what happened that has now caused the disproportionate reaction, but that would need to be done carefully with a trauma therapist.

## Body scans

It is important to carefully ask the child about their bodily sensations: their chest and heartbeat, their breathing, their head and any dizziness, their weak legs or almost missing getting to the toilet in time. They can slowly learn to notice where there is tension and then learn how to release the tension. This can help them increase in awareness, feel empowered with their own body and move from total numbness to being able to feel.

## Our nervous system

Back when I was a child, when someone was significantly impacted by a traumatic life, they would describe that person and their symptoms of distress as them 'having a nervous breakdown'. This always seemed a strange label to me as no one seemed able to explain how the nervous system is impacted by too much stress, trauma and distress, but it does make a degree of sense. It is important to explain this to children so that they can begin to look after themselves and their nervous system, just as we explain how to clean their teeth to avoid decay.

Our nervous system is best described as a massive motorway that connects our brain, spinal cord and a huge network of nerves across our body that sends millions of messages all the time. It enables us to feel emotions, move our body, think, feel pain and interact with our environment appropriately. These nerve networks receive information from inside and outside the body and decide what to do in response.

We can move into panic and back into safety within minutes according to the information that we receive. As humans, we are always sending messages to other humans and receiving them without even thinking, but we still react to those messages. Our nervous system can become overwhelmed in the short term or get stuck in overwhelm, which is where things can eventually cause really worrying behaviours, and that's probably what happened to those who were described as having a 'nervous breakdown'. Sometimes we can get muddled in what information we receive from our nervous system because we have had past experiences that cause us to form the wrong conclusions.

The nervous system can be divided into two main systems:

- The sympathetic nervous system – which controls our stress reactions and helps us react quickly when danger is perceived. It causes cortisol and adrenaline to be pumped so we can respond to the danger.
- The parasympathetic nervous system – which helps us relax, rest and digest by slowing down our heart rate and breathing.

They work in opposite ways. The sympathetic system is more like an accelerator in a car and the parasympathetic system is more like the brake. When the child has a regulated nervous system, they can easily flow between both sympathetic and parasympathetic systems.

## The polyvagal theory

Stephen Porges' (2017) theory develops this further by suggesting that the shifts in our autonomic nervous system produce three states:

- rest and digest (ventral vagal)
- fight or flight (sympathetic)
- shutdown (dorsal vagal).

When we feel comfortable and safe, we can stay in the social engagement system, which is the ventral vagal system, because we feel able to engage socially. If we feel suddenly threatened, we may move into the sympathetic nervous system, where we naturally fill with adrenaline and are ready to use our fight or flight response. But if we see danger and instantly know we can't use our fight or flight response, then we may immediately freeze, immobilize or shut down and that can become a dissociative reaction to the inability to even attempt to defend against the threat – that's the dorsal vagal response. These are the three possible reactions to what we 'sense' or 'pick up' around us or inside ourselves. We are constantly sending and receiving messages about safety and danger from and about those around us.

When children understand this, by using examples such as those in this book, they can begin to understand why they react in the ways they do. That is a huge step towards recovery.

So, what can children do to move from the sympathetic nervous system to the parasympathetic nervous system so that they can learn and play? Here are some suggestions:

- Walk outside to get some fresh air.
- Pick up a comforting object – depending on their age (teddy, drink, blanket, smelly hand cream).
- Listen to music that they have ready on a playlist.
- Imagine their safe place – with smells, sights, experiences that feel calming.
- Blow ping-pong balls with a straw as a race or do other breathing exercises.
- Do some grounding exercises such as those in Section 2 that they have practised when calm.
- Shake their arms and legs or dance.
- Sing with others.
- Use a journal to record their feelings.
- Other activities that they have explored with you when they were feeling calm and able to reflect.

If they are stuck in dorsal vagal (parasympa-thetic shutdown), they can try these strategies:

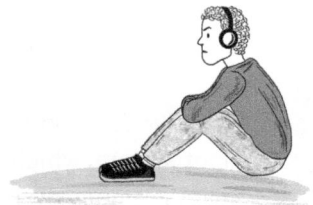

- First, start to visualize movement, any movement at all.
- Move even a little bit, such as raising an arm, stretching out an arm for a cup. Slowly move more as they begin to be able.

- Connect with someone or a pet.
- Hum or sing along gently to a familiar song.

## Neuroception

Neuroception is the automatic process of scanning the environment for risks or danger. Many children can scan an adult's face, and if they seem grumpy, they may think that the adult needs a cup of tea and so they run off with no worries. They would draw that conclusion from their own experiences of maybe their parent looking grumpy because they were thirsty. However, a child who has been hit or shouted at or punished in some other way when the adult looked grumpy may have a rather more dramatic reaction to the grumpy face and may fight, be defensive, run away, please the adult, freeze on the spot or many other possibilities. They are unable to forget the context of the face they've seen because they had an instinctive, immediate survival reaction that caused them to quickly react to stay alive. When we can explain that to traumatized children and explain that sometimes we may have what we call 'faulty neuroception', they can begin to slowly feel able to double-check their reactions in a known and safe place, so that they don't do anything quite so sudden and defensive.

I wrote a lot about this in my book *The Simple Guide to Complex Trauma and Dissociation* (2020), which is worth reading if you are keen to fully grasp the complexities of both this and the other dissociation strategies that are so little understood by even the professionals using the term. Here is a helpful quote from that book:

Sadly, we can all have a faulty neuroception, especially when we have experienced complex trauma. The nervous system is continually assessing safety or danger and reacting accordingly. For traumatized children there are so many things that remind their body or their subconscious of their unmet needs and traumatic experience that they can spend almost all of the time in a defensive state, waiting to protect themselves from the next danger. When a child assesses risk when there is none, then they can begin to create stories that can justify their evaluation, or they wear masks to help them feel defended as they continue to avoid emotional connection where they can't trust others. It can be confusing because their subconscious may detect risk based on a small factor that is no longer relevant, but the information is not cognitively available. (de Thierry, 2020, p.95)

## Interoception and depersonalization

Interoception is the process of learning to be reflective about our body and the sensations we may be feeling. When there is too much pain and body memory of past traumatic events, the child may shut down these feelings; this is called depersonalization, which is a form of dissociation. Dissociation is a way to separate some aspects of the self to stay alive in the face of unrelenting stress. Depersonalization is a way for the person to separate off some part of their body sensations to avoid total overwhelm, and it can lead to physical issues such as fainting, bladder or bowel challenges due to not being able to feel when they need to use the toilet, cutting themselves so that they feel pain and feel alive again, overeating or undereating, hurting themselves and not noticing the blood or pain, and other challenges. They may feel shame about any toileting challenges and may need support as they learn to feel those subtle signs of needing to use the bathroom. It's important to reassure them that these symptoms are a sign that they have been incredibly brave through things that never should have happened to them. One young boy told me about this symptom using the words, 'I have hard skin, I can't feel.'

How does a child recover from this? They first need to understand how clever they that are their body has worked out how to keep going when it felt overwhelmed with too many confusing or horrible memories, and then they need to slowly start to want to feel again. Again, *The Simple Guide to Complex Trauma and Dissociation* (2020) explores in far more depth the process of recovery from depersonalization and other dissociation coping mechanisms that are subconscious or unconscious strategies the child adopts to try and stay alive in the face of unrelenting terror.

It's important that we help children get stronger and more familiar with these new reflective experiences by helping them explore their reactions to simple, everyday things like the taste of chocolate or the feeling of crunchy leaves that we can stamp in. These non-threatening experiences can begin to help form familiarity and develop curiosity and then explore any emotional and/or verbal response to the feeling. Other non-threatening sensory experiences can be helpful, although we do need to be wise with some sensory activities that could trigger children with certain traumatizing backgrounds. (de Thierry, 2020, p.105)

## When their body memories are due to neglect

My book *The Simple Guide to Emotional Neglect* (2023) explores in detail how to help a child who has a history of emotional neglect recover every aspect of their body, unconscious, emotions, relationships and memory. Here are a few lines from it:

> We know that when a baby or a child is left physically on their own for any length of time it can be deeply stressful. This is different from a child choosing to withdraw and be on their own, where they feel in control. Children need to feel connected to and near an adult who can help them so that they don't feel powerless and frightened. They should experience being rocked, thrown in the air with laughter, patted and massaged in age-appropriate ways, and as they get older only with consent that is authentic. This helps them feel as if they own their own body and they can feel familiar in their own skin, rather than feeling like a stranger to themselves.
>
> When a child hasn't had enough touch and playful interactions with their body such as rocking, jumping, swinging and other such large movements, they can end up with behaviours that involve tense shoulders, holding their breath, exhaustion from holding things in, avoidance of hugs and avoidance of any other touch, which can lead to isolation and fear of connection and digestive issues from the tension. It's never too late to start to explore different soothing touch and large movement activities; as long as the child can feel 100% able to say 'no' to anything that makes them feel uncomfortable.
>
> When a child has experienced emotionally connected and attuned parenting, they are able to feel at home in their own body. They feel in control and comfortable being around other people and keeping the boundary of their body. When a child has not had that repetitive nurturing touch and soothing, they can feel shocked and unsettled if someone brushes past them, or if someone touches their shoulder.

Their body can become rigid or shut down in order to avoid processing the feelings that the touch can elicit. (de Thierry, 2023, pp.74–75)

## Other body memories and symptoms of distress and what to do for recovery

Some of the reasons that children self-harm and struggle with disordered eating are due to the distracting and painful feelings in their body and emotions which they don't know how to manage. They are using the self-harming behaviours as a way to self-medicate and manage the distress and pain. They may also be attempting to manage the consequences of symptoms such as depersonalization where they cannot access feelings easily, which can lead them to want to feel pain or discomfort or hunger so that they can feel that they are alive. What we need to realize is that when people get triggered into different defence mechanisms or coping strategies such as these, or if they find themselves shutting down in some way, they may develop elaborate narratives to make sense of what they are doing with their body, or they may not be aware of their reactions because of the shock and shame they may feel about it.

## How do children begin to heal and recover from these symptoms of distress?

Sadly, we cannot just focus on the symptoms, but instead we need to reflect on why these behaviours have in some way helped them cope better. They may feel as if they are managing their distressing feelings, which is why it can be difficult for them to stop controlling their eating or self-harming. This is usually because in the actual moment of using these coping mechanisms their lives did feel better, albeit for a short moment. So they need to be courageous enough to reflect on why they needed to do this? What bodily feelings were they avoiding feeling? What did those remind them of? Why did they so need to avoid them and how could they begin to feel safe enough to allow a tiny bit of those feelings to be felt and be validated.

If there are some memories that begin to surface, the important thing is that the adult listening or being present doesn't panic but is calm, kind, comforting, affirming and validating. The child will need a lot of support to use their voice to say what happened, because we know that it was so terrible and terrifying that they had to survive by avoiding any feeling and stopping the pain by being numb.

'I just want it to be over and I am fed up with my body memories interrupting my life. It's like I have no choice but to face what happened to me and admit it was horrific and should never have happened to a young child. Then there are lots of emotions and it's all just a lot to deal with. But I'd rather do it now than have it there like a secret that I spend my life dreading.' *James, aged 17*

## Self-harming behaviours

There has been an increase in self-harming behaviours, and research is clear that often they are used as a coping mechanism where the feeling of harm to the body alleviates feelings of emotional distress. Judith Herman (2022) says, 'Self injury is intended not to kill but rather to relieve unbearable emotional pain, and many survivors regard it, paradoxically, as a form of self-preservation' (p.109). Children who have survived significant trauma, especially from an early age, can find themselves needing to move from being numb, disorientated, frozen or dissociative to suddenly panicking and wanting to feel fully alive. An effective although destructive method to help them feel alive is to shock themselves into a state of feeling again by self-harming. Children can often live with a conflict of needing to feel numb and then needing to feel alive again. 'As one survivor explains, "I do it to prove I exist"' (Herman, 2022, p.109).

There can be a lot of other reasons for the behaviour, including social media influencing young people and it being modelled as almost a rite of passage into teenage years, or as loyalty towards someone else suffering, but the primary reason is still usually seen as distress. If you find that a child has been self-harming, your first response should be an empathetic one where you validate the child's need to find ways to self-soothe, and then you can offer support and emotional availability. If the child then grows in their ability to 'open up' and explore some of the feelings they may be having and what they have been doing, it is vital to be supportive and compassionate. Even if you are terrified of what could happen with infection or it escalating to suicidal feelings, it's important to remain calm but not unemotional, or they will assume you don't care. It's appropriate to be upset when you see someone you love in distress, and the emotional reaction should be authentic but not so intense that it takes up all the space that the child requires to have their needs met. The child then needs to be offered time to explore what is going on and what support is available, and then alternative ways of expressing distress can be explored, such as journal writing, playing music, dancing or other forms of exercise. It is important to then be consistent about checking in with them regularly, to know what is happening both with the self-harming but also with their feelings of distress. What is the cause of the distress? What trauma could they be enduring? What could be done to alleviate that in a more positive way?

If the self-harm continues, it is important to seek specialist help and to explain that this way of coping isn't really a permanent solution due to the possibility of long-term harm or infection. It is appropriate for a caring adult to seek professional help for the distressed child if the emotional connection, space to be heard, seen and validated, and compassion over the length of time haven't met the needs that may underly the symptom of distress.

## Alternatives to self-harming

The child needs to find the ways that help them the best. Everyone is different, but it's important for them to try different methods of stopping the urgent need to harm themselves, until the root reason is given the time and attention it needs. They might:

- punch a punch bag
- hold an ice cube
- draw on their arm with a red marker
- dance till they sweat
- cry, scream, shout
- call a friend
- ping an elastic band on their wrist
- apply a bandage where they want to hurt themselves
- wrap themselves in a blanket
- paint or colour
- listen to music.

## Disordered eating

When a child is struggling to feel their body and follow the natural, instinctive signals that the body gives to remind humans to eat, drink and go to the bathroom, they can end up being slower to listen to these signals. This muddled internal communication is often due to an overwhelming quantity of information that is being communicated internally regarding pain, turmoil and discomfort. The overwhelming experience of internal hidden distress can lead to some children finding comfort either in eating due to the immediate relief of any pain in their tummy or a rumbling feeling, or not eating because they don't want to feel their tummy or body. When the body is overwhelmed with trying to survive, the child can avoid eating or be restrictive in their eating as a way of coping. When they have felt powerless, being able to control an aspect of their life feels a relief and a boundary that they may want to hold strongly.

Some of the challenges around eating can be due to these reasons:

- Memories of being hungry that are held as implicit memories that drive desperation for food or familiarity of hunger.
- Memories of food being forced and the sensory and emotional panic and overload of that.
- Food being used for bribery and control, which now means that food is frightening.
- The child has depersonalization due to past trauma and so is not aware of their feelings of hunger, being full or feeling sick until it is a shock.
- Being scared when being sick or using the toilet and so they want to avoid both.
- Food seeming to be the only thing they can control in their life.
- Other experiences of choking or struggling to swallow have made them terrified.
- Food has been given by adults who seem to resent them being alive or having needs – the child learns to hide their needs and feel shame for having them.

It is recognized that eating disorders or disordered eating and dissociation are connected as survival mechanisms that are often hidden for some time and exist to help the child avoid further discomfort. They can cause additional stress to the body and mind of the child who then becomes trapped in a habit where they can feel a continual whirlwind of distress.

While the disordered eating needs to become ordered again and the depersonalized person needs to feel their body again, these symptoms are all exactly that – symptoms of distress that need to be heard, seen and validated with empathy and kindness, while the trauma experience needs to be eventually processed so that the continual internal turmoil can be resolved.

## Conclusion

When children are recovering from traumatic body memories, these are some of the things we can bear in mind.

- We can help them learn to be kind to their body that has held so much pain and stress. Help them to listen to their body and what it is trying to say rather than get annoyed with it. What area of the body hurts and what could help?
- Do they need a hot water bottle or fan, a soft blanket, calm music or a comforting drink to keep them hydrated?
- What could they do to show their body that they are grateful for it? Can they use hand cream, massage oil, eat vegetables, take up some exercise or speak kindly to themselves?
- What could they do to grow in experiencing positive touch? Who would they let stroke their head or hand, give them a back or shoulder massage or rub their feet? We know that this releases oxytocin, which decreases fear, and so can build a positive relationship with an appropriate adult while it restores something that was robbed from the child due to the trauma.
- We can help the child begin to explore what triggers their nervous system into fight/flight and what that looks like for them.
- We can explore with them what it feels like for them to feel safe enough not to stay in that state. What do they need to help them come back into their social system?
- We can also explore what habits, coping mechanisms or trauma symptoms they have now are due to coping with body memories or pains where their body was hurt through trauma. Can they

acknowledge these without shame and instead with a sense of pride that they survived?

- How can these feelings be swapped out for better ways of feeling distress? How can we help them to tolerate the feelings of distress?

There is a therapeutic book by Gabi Garcia (2017) that can help children with these issues: *Listening to My Body: A guide to helping kids understand the connection between their sensations (what the heck are those?) and feelings so that they can get better at figuring out what they need.*

## Questions to reflect on
### For parents/carers/therapeutic mentors

- What are the different automatic reactions mentioned at the start of the chapter? Which does your child use the most?
- Does your child have body memories? Do they struggle with depersonalization?
- Which of the polyvagal states does the child stay in mostly? Social engagement system or danger or threat to life?
- Do they have faulty neuroception sometimes and have reactions to things that maybe shouldn't be that frightening? What could you to do help them?
- Do they feel their body?? How can you help them feel something positive first?
- Do they struggle with eating or self-harming??

### For therapists

- What tools have you used, or could you use, to help them explore and process their body symptoms and memories?
- Has the child explored the feelings in their body, possible body memories or body discomforts?
- Are you familiar with dissociation assessment tools to explore the level of dissociative symptoms?

# CHAPTER 12

# The Impact of Trauma on the Emotions

Emotions are natural ways of expressing an experience. Each emotion is important, and no emotion is 'wrong'. In an ideal situation, the child would become confident in the process of trying to regulate their emotions in warm and caring relationships during their first five years, so that they can learn how to appropriately express emotions in a way that is not harming to themselves or others. For example, a toddler may suddenly shout, scream and throw all their food, then throw toys at the head of another child because they have finished eating their biscuit and their friend is still enjoying theirs! Their sense of frustration, jealousy, irritation, anger and injustice is not regulated but dysregulated because they are expressing exactly what they feel. When you are caring for a young toddler, it can be difficult not to laugh when this happens, because most of us recognize that we may still feel like that when something frustrates us, such as queuing for an hour for something and the person in front of us getting the last item. We may also want to scream, shout, yell and punch the ground with frustration, but we don't because we are emotionally regulated, and instead we may sigh, shed a tear and then resolve to do something positive instead, while grumbling under our breath that life sometimes sucks.

Researchers Dvir *et al.* (2014) studied the link between childhood trauma, emotional dysregulation and the progression to adult mental health challenges if the child is not supported to become regulated. They expand on the concept of regulation, explaining that emotional awareness, social cognition, the ability to recognize emotions in themselves and others and process social emotions, such as empathy, theory of mind and moral reasoning, are part of emotional regulation. These factors can help shape a perfect agenda for mentoring sessions and parenting goals.

Emotional regulation takes time to learn, and a child only learns through an adult helping them to understand how to express emotions in a positive way while giving them the language to understand what they are feeling. This is called co-regulation.

The aim of co-regulation is to help the child to:

- feel less distress
- return to a state of calm and feeling connected
- begin to learn how to self-regulate after much modelling and practising with them.

When a child experiences co-regulation, they are able to get back into 'their Window of Tolerance' and continue life with a comfortable, happy attitude. Without co-regulation, their window can grow smaller and smaller, and they spend less time feeling comfortable and more time in either hypoaroused states or hyperaroused states. A child needs to be supported relationally to be able to learn emotional regulation, and the ability to be self-regulated is seen by researchers such as Dvir *et al.* (2014) as an area of development that 'is highly influenced by the ability to develop appropriate secure attachments'. Dvir *et al.* (2014) continue by explaining that 'emotional regulation appears to develop in the context of responsive caregiving and peer involvement in early life. Not only do caregivers provide for their children's basic survival needs, but interactions with caregivers are necessary for the development of bodily self-regulation'.

## Traumatized children and their emotions

Traumatized children can feel especially terrified of their feelings because they may have internalized the big feelings of terror and powerlessness along with others such as shock, anger and confusion about why they were exposed to such terrifying things. These emotions can freeze internally and become like blocks of ice that only feel like discomfort and pain to a child who can't work out what to do with them, or they are like volcanos that spurt and spit suddenly and shock and hurt others. Their emotions need to be expressed, but slowly and carefully so that the child doesn't become further terrified by the strength and intensity of their own emotional expression. The adult needs to be prepared to be a 'container' for their overwhelming feelings and be able to 'hold them emotionally' and reflect to them what they feel is going on in a way that is comforting and reassuring. Research confirms the benefit of focusing on children understanding and expressing emotions because 'helping children recognize and express emotions can reduce the possibility of behaviour problems in adolescence and adulthood' (Li, 2023).

This is what a therapist would do, but is also something that someone who has enough experience can facilitate, and it is essential that a primary caregiver learns to naturally talk about and explain emotions to those they are looking after.

'I wish I understood that when a child is often grumpy, they could be sad. I thought I needed to tell him to get a better attitude and sort himself out. I had no idea that actually he needed my help to listen to his worries and care for him. That would have stopped the grumpiness. Instead, I told him off because I just didn't know what I do now.' *A mum*

## A home with frozen emotions

Some children grow up so afraid of feeling their emotions, let alone expressing them, because they haven't seen emotional regulation modelled and instead have only witnessed the repression or suppression of emotions. When children grow up in homes where there is a general flatness of emotional expression, with few highs or lows, they can feel unfamiliar with others who are able to express a wide range of emotions. They can be afraid of expressing anything that seems to break the silence and steadiness of a calm and quiet environment, and this can cause them to feel that they don't really belong or fit into that space because they may feel that they have a volcano of emotions inside them. It is important for children to see adults expressing a range of emotions; when they see these, they can then learn the names of the emotions and become familiar with them.

Some children are taught to override their natural feelings to 'be brave, 'be strong' and 'pull themselves together' or distract themselves, which causes the child usually to feel a disconnection to that adult and confused about how they feel and what they should feel. It is important to remember that as adults we need to help children to feel emotions. Levine and Kline (2017) beautifully explain that if children can 'learn to tolerate emotional pain in small doses, and realize that if they do, it won't last forever, they have learned one of life's most valuable lessons' (p.228).

## Experiencing the range of emotions and learning the names

Ideally, children should be able to learn emotions such as excitement, nervousness, fear, anger, frustration, annoyance, jealousy, irritation, joy, disgust, happiness, confusion and boredom, and be able to use language to describe these because they have had adults use those words during any expression of that emotion. When an adult is too fast to stop the child's emotional expression by either distracting them or telling them to stop the behaviour, emotion or words, they never get to understand what it feels like to feel the feeling and work through it to a sense of resolution. Dan Siegel (2012) coined the phrase 'name it to tame it' when describing the power of naming the emotions to bring about a sense of relief. When a child can name the feelings and use words, it helps to calm the nervous system by using the left brain's power to soothe the right brain's overwhelm. Writing in a journal or talking can be helpful for this exact process.

When adults distract the child from their feelings, it can be due to their own unresolved trauma because they don't want children in their world to experience negative feelings and they want to protect them from those. That ends up being unhelpful because they will undoubtedly experience them at some point, and it is best that they do so with a loving and caring adult who can help them know what they are feeling and what to do with those feelings. It is important to let them express an emotion, then comfort them, while explaining that they may be feeling 'x' (the name of the emotion); then in the comfort, reassurance and validation, they can be encouraged to be less loud or wild or interruptive to others. This boundary work is important along-side the comfort, so that they grow up understanding what is healthy and what is important to regulate for others' sake.

If, for example, they are screaming with terror as they get ready for a medical examination or operation, it is important to let them express the scream and then give validation, reassurance and kindness, but it also could be that distracting them from that feeling is essential for them to be able to go ahead with the important procedure. After the operation, when the child is no longer terrified and is feeling coura-geous and relieved, it could be a good time to revisit the emotional expression and, with empathy, use words to describe what the feeling looked like and how painful it was to see such fear and powerlessness. As you describe your reaction to their fear, it builds that sense of them feeling seen, heard and validated, which strengthens your relationship with them.

Currently, an extraordinary number of children are needing to have extra time in school learning this emotional language due to not having the natural relational learning that should happen in the years before they start school.

## Attuning to the child's emotions

Having first modelled that emotions are helpful indicators and are welcome to be expressed, it's important then to co-regulate their emotional expression by essentially lending our thinking and rational brain to them while they feel overwhelmed and unable to think clearly. As we articulate what we think is going on for them, they can feel reassured that we as the adult have the strength and capacity to guide them through and can help them know when to stay with the emo-tion and when to distract themselves and plan to reflect later. When children feel that their emotions are welcomed, they often need less space and time to express them because they aren't fighting to be heard and validated and they are getting what they need faster. They tend to move faster through the emotions when they feel that the adult has attuned to their needs and cares and the adult's face, tone of voice and body language communicate this. Sometimes they need to know that the adult cares about their distress more than how they are perceived by other adults.

## Our own fear of emotions

Often the reason that the child can be dysregulated with their emotions is because the adults around them may be terrified or feel too exposed or vulnerable about their own emotions. Maybe you have bottled up your own feelings and tried to bury them so that you can keep going and not end up exploding or imploding. It's important for all the adults to go on their own journey of exploration of emotions and learn to slowly feel some of the emotions that may feel so deep, raw or volatile. Having someone to help you is important, so that you can safely feel and have those feelings validated and not become unstable because of the expression of them. It could be that sometimes you feel 'outside yourself' or 'beside yourself' with emotions. It could be important to learn the simple skill of being still, hearing your breath, noticing the sensations in your body – maybe your chest feeling tight or your head spinning or your tummy feeling tension – and as you feel these, you can carefully ground yourself to the present by noticing some things around you that bring calm and comfort, remembering that you are not powerless now and your feelings will not overwhelm you completely. Then you can validate your own emotions and be kind to yourself as you are navigating this path. You may find that you let out a big breath or need to find a cushion to hug, or you cry. Sit with these feelings and don't minimize them or be ashamed of them. The value you bring to this moment is important and can enable you to respond to the child with more authenticity as you have walked the same path.

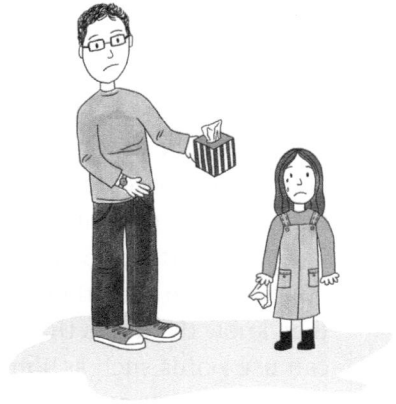

## Emotional language to support the child

The first step is to try and help them label the emotion. Don't tell them what it is but use the language around 'I'm wondering if you feel...' This enables them to disagree with you. It's never about who is right and who is wrong, but instead it is about building a culture where they can learn to reflect and be curious about their emotions before they explode or implode! When they are brave enough to suggest that they may be feeling something, it's important that the adults validate those feelings with empathy and use language such as 'I'm sorry that you feel like that, but well done for letting me know' or 'It's okay to feel that because of how that person took your pen' or 'I'm sure many people would feel like that if that had happened to them'. These words help the child feel accepted and that their emotion is acknowledged, which helps them to continue to explore their feelings.

It is important when this is happening to keep in mind the need for boundaries to keep them safe so that when they express an emotion, they know the limits that they would need in different contexts. You can use words such as 'I'm glad you could express that distress here where it is safe to scream because other children aren't around who may be scared' or 'It's important that you express the anger you feel about what happened here with me so that you can be calm with your friends now and enjoy playing'. Emotions need boundaries, and adults need to help the child understand that as they learn to express and explore them. The child will need to have time to reflect on how the emotional expression made them feel, what happened to their body and their mind, how much more they feel needs to be expressed and how else they could express the feelings. This can lead to reflecting on ideas for further expression alongside ideas for how to safely and appropriately express emotion in other settings such as in school or at a party.

## When a child is stuck in overwhelm or shock

It's important to assess shock by noticing the physical appearance of the child and assessing their breathing, heart rate, eyes and if the pupils are dilated. Do they look vacant, zoned out, as if they are not present in their own body, or are they confused or screaming irrationally? When someone has had a shock, they often don't feel the physical pain and haven't grasped what has happened, because the body is clever and the instinctive reaction to threat can serve as a natural analgesia to stop any feelings of pain. This means that they should not be left on their own so that they can be kept safe.

If they are shocked, it's important to stay calm and confident, to reassure them and validate them and any emotions they may be expressing. As the adult, you need to speak and communicate clearly what it is happening and what you are going to do – this is when internalized thinking can cause further distress. Your words of reassurance and confidence that safety can be found and things will be better soon are essential. Sometimes the child may shake or become cold, and it's important to let them shake as that is a natural reaction following terror. Helping them become warm is important, so they feel nurtured and cared for.

## Anger

The emotion that is often hardest to work with and has the biggest impact on others around them is anger. Anger has a purpose and is often essential for the child to be able to protect themselves and express some of the pain and turmoil in a way that involves less vulnerability than sadness. It is not 'wrong' for the child to feel anger and it's important to explore that with a child, until they realize that there is a valid reason for feeling the injustice, helplessness and frustration of what happened to them. They often need their feelings of anger validated as a reasonable reaction to the loss and pain of the trauma or as sadness that has few words.

Sometimes children do focus their anger on their parents or carers, and this can, of course, cause pain and distress, which can escalate the challenges of supporting them through to recovery. It is important to try and remember that even when the anger seems personal, it may not be, but may instead be deep sadness at lots of factors that need time and space to explore.

However, many people associate anger with violence, and that can escalate relational dynamics as those around the child can become fearful for their own safety. Therefore, it is important for the child to be able to release the anger in a way that is not violent or destructive. The stage before that would be to help the child recognize the connection between a trauma experience and their feelings of anger. Music (2019) highlights that 'aggression from the Latin literally means to "move forwards", a positive trait, the opposite of shrinking' (p.33), and therefore to some extent, if it is supported to be expressed in a way that doesn't harm another person, it can be a helpful release. The expression and release of the feeling can also bring a sense of relief as things begin to make sense. The child will also begin to see a decrease in somatic symptoms that often accompany unexpressed anger, such as tummy aches, headaches, digestive difficulties and others.

Here are the steps to help a child with their anger:

- Give the child ways to release anger that are helpful.
- Help them feel the feeling and then express it.
- Help them to use words as they express their anger so that they know why they are expressing it.
- Explain what anger is, and explore what makes them angry and what they can do when they feel that.

Some children need to be supported in finding an appropriate way to release the anger that they feel. They can explore how others may be frightened by the expression of it, and so finding healthy ways to release it is important. Here are some ideas for releasing anger:

- Exercise of some kind – running, boxing or other movement.
- Trampoline games and movement.
- Throwing clay or newspaper that has been soaked in water.
- Throwing or trying to smash ice.
- Writing down the angry words on a large piece of paper.
- Creating a dance or haka that expresses defensive moves.

## A healthy relationship with emotions

These times of expressing emotion should lead to a more confident relationship with emotions, knowing what words can be used to describe them and what the child can do another time to express them in a healthy way. It should lead them to understand the nature of emotions and what happens when humans don't express them but lock them up inside. They should understand how to express emotions that feel overwhelming and explosive in a safe way that makes their insides feel less like a volcano. It is important that we help children to have a good relationship with their emotions where they recognize that 'feelings come and go. They are noticed, they are responded to, they are processed as they arise. They don't get stuck' (Gerhardt, 2004, p.198).

## Conclusion

The traumatized child will often have dysregulated emotions that seem far too huge to begin to feel or express. They do, however, need to be expressed and validated, held and acknowledged for trauma recovery to take place. The consequence of having an adult able to co-regulate their emotions is that they become more able to be emotionally literate and intelligent. This co-regulation, alongside them also feeling less weighed down with unexpressed or frozen emotions, is one of the less painful elements of the journey towards trauma recovery.

## Questions to reflect on
### For parents/carers/therapeutic mentors

- What emotional expression from a child causes you to be distressed? What could you do to allow the expression of it but with healthy boundaries, so you don't get hurt or too overwhelmed?
- Have you got experience with an environment that doesn't allow emotional expression and yet you sense a lot of the people who are there have unexpressed, big emotions that seem to rumble? What do you feel like?
- Do you feel afraid of emotional expression? What could you do?
- What range of emotions do you express, and do you use language to name these emotions?
- Have you witnessed an explosion or implosion of emotions in the child you are caring for? What could you have done to support this person?
- Have you been stuck in overwhelm or cared for a child who has? What have you done to help them become less stuck?

### For therapists

- Are you using the Window of Tolerance with children to help them notice where they are in or near the window?
- Which emotion that a child or parent/carer expresses causes you the most challenge, resistance or lack of focus, and what have you done or could you do to ensure attunement?

# CHAPTER 13

# The Subconscious and Unconscious

The area of the subconscious and unconscious seems to be the one that has the least attention in the fast-growing interest in trauma recovery at present. Years ago, it was seen as the primary area of impact to be addressed. It is the area that is most complex but arguably the most essential to understand, certainly with complex trauma.

Trauma impacts the nervous system and the body, and there is continual growing research that helps us know what to do to help bring back health and calm. The impact of trauma on emotions and relationships is also an area that is relatively clear and can be written about with some simplicity, although some ideas are harder to practise in the context of real in-person emotionally intense or exhausting relationships! The known mind and our thoughts are an area that has had a lot of attention over the decades, and many health services offer simple cognitive or verbal therapies to help. However, it is the unconscious and subconscious areas of our mind that hold a lot of the complex coping mechanisms and defence mechanisms that are invisible in many ways but cause the most confusion to the traumatized person and those trying to support them. It is this area that is the main reason why many of the resources and provision for traumatized children are not fully working. It is causing children to believe that they are 'too broken', when they just need professionals who are trained effectively to help them.

## The volatility of the subconscious and unconscious
The unconscious is the area that functions below the area of the known conscious, outside awareness. This area is often not the point of focus

for many practitioners, including those who say they are trauma recovery specialists, and so the child who is being supported may make good progress in their emotional regulation, trust with supporting adults and emotional literacy. They may become confident in exercises and movements that strengthen areas of the brain and body that could have held stress, shock, tension or been underdeveloped due to developmental trauma that occurred in the child's first five years. The child may be supported to be able to do some difficult tasks and use language to explain what they need and how they feel. However, they also may behave in ways that seem to shock them, where they suddenly react dramatically to a big noise or to a situation that they seemed fine about the day before. The child may be normal one moment and then suddenly 'become an animal', or have no memory of the previous day or hour. They may be calm one moment and then in the next may shout, yell, kick and throw furniture at you. They may then have no memory of doing so. They might suddenly speak about suicidal thoughts where there was no indicator of such thinking before.

The volatility is because the child has unprocessed memories and trauma experiences that are not held as conscious memories, and these memories can interrupt them with reactions that seem to make no sense to them or anyone else. This is usually due to the subconscious or unconscious mind that needs to be carefully facilitated in being able to slowly process what has happened.

## Why can't they talk about what happened?

There is a good reason why many adults don't disclose abuse or other trauma for decades. It felt too unsafe and the possibility of what lay in the dark recesses of the soul were too terrifying and they didn't really want to know and didn't want to think anything had happened. Our clever mind allows us to push things down so far that we cannot remember, or only a part of us can remember only a snippet of what happened. That shard of memory can just feel like a splinter that is there and is uncomfortable, but unless you press on it or focus on it, you can mostly pretend it's not there. Children are the same. They may remember that they absolutely *hate* the smell of smoke or attics but have no idea what led to that passionate opinion.

## Moving things from the unconscious mind to the conscious mind

What we know about the unconscious mind is that it is the part of us that has unprocessed experiences in it that have led to beliefs and opinions, and that it informs us what is safe and dangerous and can influence more of our behaviour and thinking than we like to think. Carl Jung (1973) says that 'man's task is to become conscious of the contents that press upward from the unconscious'. The job of moving experiences and memories from the unconscious to the conscious needs careful consideration and training. In Chapter 16 on trauma processing, we explore creating an integrative narrative, but this needs to be a slow and steady process once other aspects of recovery have been established. For the child survivor, it is not fun, enjoyable or pleasant to move memories and experiences from the unconscious mind to the conscious mind. It takes courage and commitment.

*This area of the brain is so complex that if someone 'has a go' at helping but hasn't been trained and clinically supervised by someone who is very experienced, it could lead the child to become destabilized and far more volatile. It is a delicate area that needs careful reflection to be able to help the child move towards healing rather than further stress, chaos, fragmentation and increased defence mechanisms.*

The unconscious is the area of the mind that holds the unprocessed feelings, thoughts, relational experiences, sensory experiences, shocking experiences and emotions. Before the child can talk about it or tell anyone what happened and simultaneously feel the emotions that are appropriate to feel when they speak of the experience, the unconscious needs to become conscious. If all these unprocessed memories become conscious immediately, it would probably cause the child to implode, because the reason that the memories are not in the conscious mind and readily available to them in their here and now is that it would cause them to feel completely overwhelmed, terrified and powerless. It was 'too much' when they first experienced these things, and so they had to be pushed down for processing when they were able. A child who is imploding is usually one who escalates quickly into cycles of panic, distress and either anger or silence, and where they consequently often begin to no longer function with the daily challenges that a child must complete, such as toileting, washing, eating, drinking and taking part in group activities, without a lot of support. Now these children may need one-to-one attention a lot of the time or they withdraw and seem to give up on the effort of human relationships due to living in an overwhelmed state.

*To get a child to talk about all that's happened to them and how they feel is like asking them to take every paper document in a filing cabinet and throw them on the floor along with all the toys on the shelves and all the food in the cupboard, and then be pleased that we've made the unconscious conscious!*

We need to avoid children imploding or exploding. Therefore, we need to make sure that the professionals working with the child in this area are working with clinical supervisors and have had specific training in the complexity of the unconscious, because trying to help a child's psyche process trauma experiences too quickly and without an understanding of the sequential order of externalizing that which is currently in the unconscious can be unhelpful or dangerous. Let's explore some of the things that happen in the unconscious so we can tread carefully and respect the coping mechanisms that humans can use automatically to survive.

## Denial, repression and suppression

Repression is the coping mechanism that enables a person to unconsciously keep difficult information, memories and experiences from their conscious mind; suppression is the conscious decision to do the same. Denial is a word more commonly used to describe both those processes. It is a commonly understood coping mechanism, which can be conscious or unconscious, known or not known in the cognitive mind. We can use denial when we feel a sense of shame or awkwardness over what we've just said or done and it feels too overwhelming to process in the moment. We can sometimes realize we are using denial, such as eating a chocolate bar which we know we shouldn't eat that day, but we eat it while saying we are in denial and soon after we can pretend that we didn't eat it. We remain able to know that we did eat it, but we are trying to play tricks on our own mind to forget.

When there is trauma involved, denial can be used as an unconscious coping mechanism because the mind seems to sweep away the memory in urgency to protect the person from being too overwhelmed by the horrors of the experience. The visual memory, sensory memory and emotional memory can be pushed down quickly in an instinctual urgent desire to never remember what just happened. That can enable someone to keep going in a terrifying situation, such as being able to run away or carry on and finish their work for the day. Later in the day, the memory may begin to come towards the surface of the conscious, and the person can either choose to push it down again or allow it to bubble up. The issue again here is that if someone has had to use denial to get through a situation, when they do then remember the experience, it may cause shock or terror, and that can be overwhelming because they can also feel shame about why they seemed to forget something so horrific. Silberg (2012) affirms that 'self-protective memory processes help clients avoid thinking of painful events, and soon the child survivors may no longer remember what happened to them' (p.180).

## The basic neurobiology of memory

The 'middle' area of the brain is called the limbic system, and it is in this area where the amygdala and hippocampus work together with each other around our memory and emotions. They have very different roles to aid in the retrieval of memories and the storing of them. The amygdala is often referred to as the fear centre because it is primarily responsible for the emotional content of memories and acts as a warning system for the brain and body by scanning the environment for potential threats. The hippocampus is essential for long-term memory, and it's this area of the brain that has been evidenced to show shrinkage when childhood trauma has happened (Vythilingam *et al.*, 2002). It is the part of the brain that helps specific memories fit within the context of other previous life experiences. It also links together other sensory experiences that occurred during the traumatic experience, such as sights, sounds and smells.

## What do you do if the child is in denial?

As an adult supporting a child who has experienced trauma, it is essential to try and notice the facial reactions and nervous system shifts of a child when they are talking about something that happened to them. If they look shocked, you can guess that

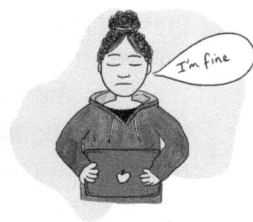

they didn't really know before they said it using their own voice, and now they wish they hadn't heard those words and could go back into denial again. It's obviously important not to stare or look too intently, but looking to grasp a sense of what is happening with their stress response system is vital so that they can have help gently to come out of denial and be greeted with nurture, validation and care, and all with an emphasis on them not being to blame. Denial is used day to day in useful ways, but it is also a lifesaving tool for many people who cannot acknowledge, accept or process what happened as it was too overwhelming. Researchers looking at childhood trauma survivors noted that 'some deny their trauma history' (Crummy & Downey, 2022).

It can be traumatizing for a child to be told to come out of denial and face the facts, and it can be deeply distressing for them to be told what happened to them if they are saying it didn't. Adults need a lot of wisdom and emotional skills to be able to help a child have the right emotional foundations in place to hear some of the stories of what happened to them. Section 1 explores these foundations that need to be in place before it is safe to unpack that which they have 'filed away'. The child probably has a sense of what happened but doesn't want it confirmed – and yet they do want it confirmed. That conflict can be intense and can cause enormous emotional meltdowns and stress for them. It's essential for the child to feel in control of the process of their own story, and when and if they ask for some information, it's important to let them know a bit at a time so they can stop whenever they need to. The child will probably reply to any questions with 'I'm fine' and 'Honestly, it's okay' to avoid the feeling of vulnerability and exposure that can be terrifying. For a child who has experienced trauma, it can be horrific to remember elements of what happened, and they can feel stuck between the painful conflict that the 'denial of reality makes them feel crazy, but acceptance of the full reality seems beyond what any human being can bear' (Herman, 1998, p.181).

It is also important to know that often a child has a sense of fear that they will be accused of lying about what happened. They are often told they are liars, and so the fear of being accused of that while being courageous enough to speak about some of what they experienced can grip them. They can hear whispers of 'you've made it up' and 'you're exaggerating' and 'you just want attention', which can cause them to be silent or assume they did make it up.

## Dissociation

It is vital to understand that it is impossible to help children who have experienced Type III trauma and a lot of Type II trauma recover without an understanding of how to help someone who has dissociation as a coping mechanism. Often when therapy 'isn't working', it is because dissociation hasn't been noticed, understood or acknowledged. Here is a short extract from *The Simple Guide to Complex Trauma and Dissociation* which covers this subject in greater depth:

> Dissociation is a way of separating or distancing in order to survive. It is a biological survival mechanism and a psychological defence system. Putnam says, 'dissociation is often conceptualized as a defensive process that protects the individual in the face of overwhelming trauma' (1997, p.75). A person can experience being disconnected from themselves, including their memories, feelings, actions, thoughts, body and even their identity. For some people, this could be a short-term survival strategy that is useful to survive a crisis but then is not used again, but in this book, we want to explore the coping mechanism that can persist for months, years, or a lifetime and often way past when it was needed for survival. For many children they not only dissociate during the traumatic event but then any time they are reminded about that event. Dissociation can allow the person to compartmentalize and disconnect from aspects of traumatic experiences that could otherwise overwhelm their capacity to cope. It enables the traumatic memories to be kept far away from the core self but becomes a dysfunctional coping mechanism that causes all sorts of problems. (de Thierry, 2020, pp.50–51)

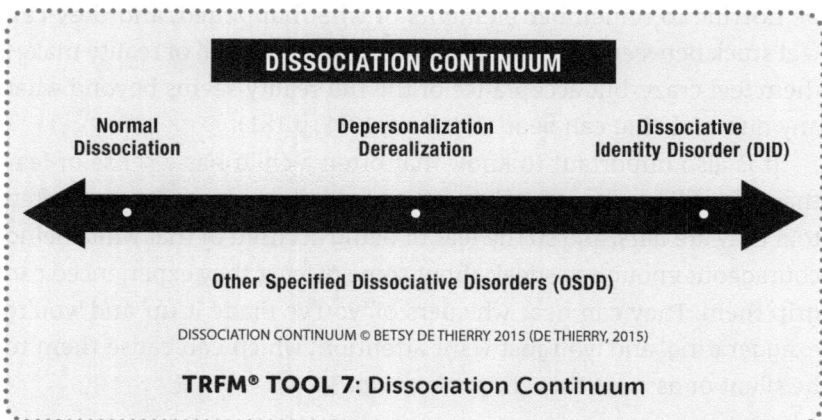

**DISSOCIATION CONTINUUM**

| Normal Dissociation | Depersonalization Derealization | Dissociative Identity Disorder (DID) |

Other Specified Dissociative Disorders (OSDD)

DISSOCIATION CONTINUUM © BETSY DE THIERRY 2015 (DE THIERRY, 2015)

**TRFM® TOOL 7**: Dissociation Continuum

The Dissociation Continuum shows the difference in severity of symptoms from those which society is mostly familiar with, such as zoning out or spacing out a bit, towards the middle of the continuum where the person has now separated an element of themselves so that they can survive. Depersonalization is when a person subconsciously separates out their body and body sensations from the rest of themselves, usually due to overwhelming experiences in the body which are now painful body memories. This dissociative symptom could have formed due to many different experiences, such as serious medical trauma where the child's body was being hurt, or abuse or ongoing hunger. This symptom can lead to many other symptoms which can be interruptive to their life, such as challenges with toileting, eating, noticing when they are hurt and so being able to get help, and not noticing other signs of danger or pain. Depersonalization is explored further in Chapter 11. Derealization is when the child separates from their mind to escape the horrors of the trauma. They may describe being 'over their body' or 'flying above their own body' or they may 'go somewhere' more beautiful in their mind, which can then become an instant reaction to stress or terror. This can lead to disclosures using language that seems to describe 'what happened to the body', almost as if it wasn't them. Some children describe 'going to' places of safety, weapon-making factories, islands that are beautiful or settings that seem like online game scenes in their mind.

The furthest end of the continuum is when the person has fragmented into many parts due to the level of pain and turmoil they have experienced, either from terrifying things happening to them or the lack of emotional connection that comes from emotional neglect. A lack of emotional connection can lead to a child being traumatized and dissociating, so this trauma symptom may impact the child who has enough food and drink, toys and screens but does not have 'enough' emotional connection with an adult where they feel listened to, known, seen, understood, supported, validated and emotionally 'held', and so they internalize and fragment to survive what feels terrifying.

## Dissociation and parts

Again, this subject is covered at length in my book *The Simple Guide to Complex Trauma and Dissociation*, but so you can decide if it could be an area that is the main symptom or challenge for the recovery of the child you are caring for, here is a taster of the theories I have created about it.

The important element is that I don't believe anyone wants to have dissociative parts and it should not become a major element of their identity, but rather the sign that they have survived experiences that were horrific, and they now need support to recover from the impact of those years of their life. Recovery and healing are the lens that I use to approach this subject.

## The VIP theory

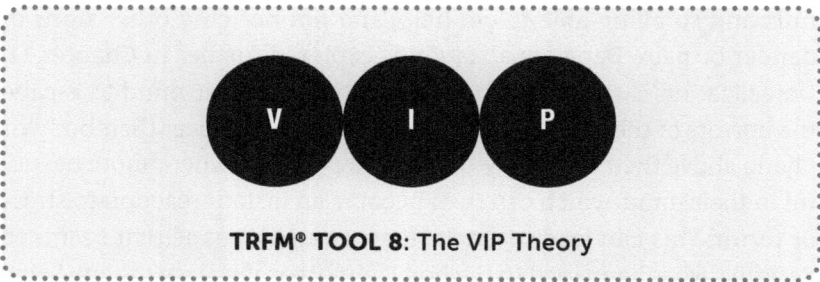

TRFM® TOOL 8: The VIP Theory

I explain that the idea that humans are as simple as that which we can see and comprehend is inefficient and unhelpful. We all recognize that when we read books like this or attend training on the subject, we cannot help but dart in our minds from reflecting on the child(ren) that we are professionally caring for, to thoughts of our own childhood experiences and those who we love. I describe that as being a VIP. We are three parts in one: we have our vulnerable part which is the part of us that builds emotionally intimate relationships, falls in love and feels rejection and abandonment deeply. We are also able to be professional and reflect on our role and keep our vulnerabilities hidden from where it would be inappropriate to share. We also have an inner child that may be happy and healthy and is therefore playful and fun to be around, or it may be jealous of the children who are getting the help they need and is stuck in survival and hidden on the inside of us, away from anyone else's view or sighting. When we react to something that happens in our world, we may have a combination of reactions that sometimes conflict as we struggle to offer professional help, while feeling turmoil in empathy for those who have endured the trauma; it may be similar to an experience we have endured, and our inner child may want to hide, scream, cry or be driven to fix it or stop it happening again.

It could be that your workplace explores the possibility of a promotion and you feel an inner conflict between your professional part that feels it is about time you were noticed and recognized for your skill, your vulnerable part that fears the possibility of failure or public humiliation, and your inner child, which may be dreaming of a new car and holidays and looking forward to seeing themselves as important and powerful so they can be less scared of powerlessness.

When people can understand themselves like this, it normalizes some of the inner conflict that can occur during difficulties or on a day-to-day basis. When we can explain that to children, it helps them understand how they can have their special blanket at home (inner child), and they can explore their trauma experiences with some grown-ups (vulnerable), but it's best to be age appropriate so that they can enjoy peer relationships (professional). Being in any specific 'part' does not deny the existence of the other.

This is not describing dissociative parts, however; instead, it is more like viewing the person from three different angles as you would a bottle of wine – from the label, the bird's-eye view and the bottom. It's the same bottle, just different angles!

## The daisy theory

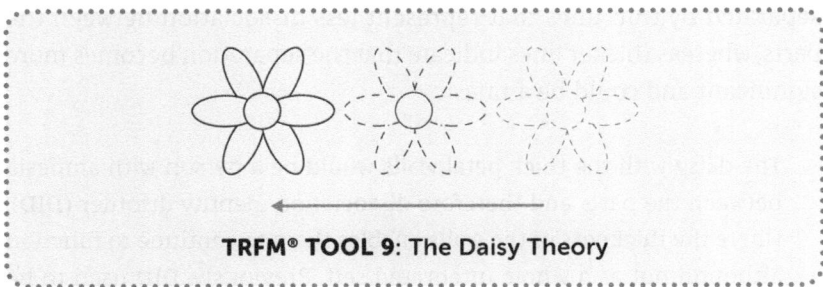

**TRFM® TOOL 9**: The Daisy Theory

The daisy theory, however, builds on the VIP theory to easily explore the different parts that a person may have internally, both dissociative and not. I use it to help children explore their 'dissociative system', which is essentially a way to cope with unrelenting traumatic experiences that are significantly too much for a child to cope with without some internal mechanisms that help them survive. Parts aren't symptoms and every dissociative part has a purpose and reason to exist. Each part was created to enable the child to survive something that was essentially unsurvivable, and as such, each part has a lot that needs to be expressed and communicated. The aim of therapy is not just to 'get rid of all the parts' but to recognize their role, their story and their need until it's possible that they aren't needed anymore. A lot of parts may have memories of experiences that happened when the child was very young and even preverbal.

The long-term, deeply misunderstood trauma symptom of dissociation is more common than many believe and yet few people are sufficiently trained to be able to offer recovery help.

The daisy theory helps humans explore the different 'parts' of who they are, both dissociative and not dissociative. The continuum begins from the right side where the 'petals' are not separated by dissociation but represent non-dissociative parts or angles of a person. In the middle there is some kind of dissociative separation between the parts and by the end, on the left, the child is separated with a level of amnesia about their different parts.

This theory is one that I have developed in my work with children and families to explain the way that a dissociative child has learned to cope with their traumatizing experience. In line with a psychological theory called the Watkins and Watkins Ego State Model, which is often referred to as the 'dissociation pie' model (1979), the petals are separated by thin lines that represent less dissociation between the parts, whereas thicker lines indicate that the separation becomes more significant and could be amnesic.

The daisy with the thick petal walls would be a person with amnesia between the parts and therefore dissociation identity disorder (DID), where the thickness of the walls enables them to continue to function although not as a whole integrated self. Previously, DID used to be called multiple personality disorder (MPD). The daisy model enables people to understand the dissociative continuum with ease... As the trauma and the pain increase, so the walls can become thicker and therefore the amnesia is greater between the parts: 'When trauma is such that dissociation becomes more extreme, the lines between the ego states thicken' (Wieland, 2011, p.19).

If someone has dissociative identity disorder, they would experience different parts, petals, buckets or personalities controlling their thoughts and behaviour at different times.

- They may feel like they are several different people with different opinions and memories
- They may feel like they don't have control over when these parts take over.
- They may refer to themselves as having different names and others may refer to them using different names.
- They may feel like there are huge internal conflicts, opinions and even different voices going on inside their head which can make even simple decisions hard.
- They may struggle to remember some incidents or periods of time.
- They may feel like there is something seriously wrong with them and be panicking about that.
- They may feel like they are different from their peers and may be desperate to fit in.
- They may feel constantly confused about being blamed for behaviours they cannot remember and feeling in internal turmoil. (de Thierry, 2020, pp.68–70)

It is entirely possible that the child may be completely unaware of how they present with different voices, ages or genders. They may only be aware of blanks in their memory, not knowing how they got to a particular place or where a chunk of time went. They can be very shocked to find out they presented so differently at other times and may even not believe others who tell them what they did or said. If what I have written here sounds familiar, then I suggest you get my small book that explores this specifically and then come back to this book armed with that specific knowledge. You will need that to facilitate recovery and be able to find a therapist who can effectively help the child you are caring for.

## Lying, memory confusion and temporary amnesia

As has been explored in this chapter, memory is more complex than many would understand. The current criminal justice system depends on a narrative of a traumatic event that is detailed, in order and with appropriate emotional reaction, yet that is rarely how memory works when the trauma experience is extreme. The emotional reaction can take years to be unlocked from that freeze-frame of time and the words can be hard to say and terrifying to hear said. The story of what happened often becomes fragmented as snippets or whole memories of words that were spoken, the visual images, their body sensations, the smells, the sounds, their emotions, and the absolute terror gripping the body, the mind, the voice and the breath of the person who struggles to defend themselves.

This can cause the child to not remember past events or only remember aspects of past events. They may stare blankly or look confused if they are asked what happened. If a child is hit by another child in the playground and then attempts to run away, and they are caught and taken to a room to reflect on why they ran, they may well be experiencing either total numbness or shock, or they may have a whirling in their mind of many different experiences when they were hit or held captive or felt unable to defend themselves, and so they sit silently and may be called 'naughty'. They may choose to lie about what happened, even if they end up taking the blame, because they would rather get out of the trapped feeling of an adult forcing them to think about what happened when their mind is whirling and their body is pumping adrenaline. They may have no words or no memory or a confused memory of what took place. Waters (2016) explains that 'stress can lead to the deactivation of certain critical structures in the brain that encode and consolidate memories into the conscious memory system, accounting for memory problems and dissociative responses (Brenner 2005; Perry 2001; Vermetten *et al.*, 2006)' (p.15).

When we see our unconscious like the muddy buckets in my Tool 1 (Chapter 1), then we can visualize that the more traumatic experiences end up going into the unseen muddy bucket. The more memories there are, the more they can cause overwhelm, which leads to difficulty in speaking about them, ordering them and making sense of them without kind, gentle and experienced help.

'As memories came back my head felt fuzzy, tears were always coming from nowhere, everyone around me felt louder and harsher and
I wished desperately that it wasn't true. What if I made it up? Why
would I make it up?' *Freddie, aged 14*

## Flashbacks

When any age of person experiences a traumatic event that is too
hard to immediately process and make sense of, the memories that
get 'pushed' down into the unconscious can come back suddenly when
there is a sensory trigger. They can cause reactions that seem to 'come
from nowhere' but are usually due to a sensory experience that caused
the unconscious to assume that they are unsafe, because the person
has a sudden visual or sensory memory of a past trauma that seems
as if it is happening now. Flashbacks are confusing, disorientating and
deeply inconvenient. Silberg (2012) explains that flashbacks keep coming back 'because the brain is giving the child a warning – something
you experienced in the past could come back and harm you again'
(p.200). When the child is convinced that they won't experience that
terror again, they will continue to have these warnings.

Here is a classic story that I created for my training and have used
for decades:

Ten-year-old Robert was walking his dog one day while drinking a
banana milkshake, when suddenly a car crashed into the pavement
and ran over his foot. A stranger called an ambulance and Robert was
treated for a broken foot. In the lunch hall at school, many months
later, Robert was happily getting his lunch and chatting to friends, when
someone accidentally spilt their banana milkshake on him. Robert then
screamed as if the car was crushing his foot again, flung his lunch tray
onto the floor, curled into a ball and let out blood-curdling screams.
(de Thierry, 2016, p.32)

This story illustrates how the smell of banana milkshake suddenly
caused a series of other sensory body memories that were attached to
the past traumatic experience. Whenever a child has a 'disproportionate
reaction' to a minor event or experience, we can be curious about what
other memory crashed into the mind of the child and caused confusion

and further terror. The child can only 'stop' the flashbacks by being able to process and make sense of the past traumas that are coming back to them. This cannot be rushed and needs to be carefully handled so that the child is given a safe, unrushed space to build emotional connection and safety with a trained adult who knows how to gently guide them through the trauma experience in a way that doesn't destabilize them or cause them to implode.

When a flashback occurs or when a memory begins to surface, it can feel as if the memory is a dream or someone else's story. It can feel silent, without emotion or sound, and therefore like something that happened to someone else. It can take a long time for a survivor to realize that it is their own memory and that they have tried to forget and deny it, but it is bubbling to the surface to be processed. This can cause things to feel as if they are slowing down, or for the person to panic as if it is happening again. It is part of the trauma recovery journey and can feel full of pain and turmoil, and so the child will need emotional support and reassurance that they haven't made up the memories or parts of the memories and that what happened should not have happened to them.

## Night terrors and nightmares

These are like flashbacks but happen while the child is asleep. It is recognized that during sleep the mind naturally processes experiences and sorts and 'files' them during the REM (rapid eye movement) stage. Dan Siegel describes the REM sleep process as 'one where looking first left and then right activates both hemispheres of the brain repeatedly'. He also describes this process as 'necessary for the consolidation and organization of memory' (Gomez-Perales, 2015, p.27).

Night terrors and nightmares can be distressing and disorientating, and again the biggest issue is that the child can struggle to comprehend them as being in the past when they feel so real and are so interruptive of the safety of their sleep. It is helpful to explain to the child what happens when we sleep and how we process our day and our experiences, and how sometimes they get muddled in our minds. Using the muddy bucket analogy can help them be keen to spend time processing some of their past experiences so that they don't interrupt them at night. The bedroom may now not feel safe because of the interruption of the memories, and so new sensory reminders of safety need to be added to help them feel secure.

While the child is on a trauma recovery journey, it is not unusual for the nightmares to increase rather than decrease, and therefore preparations need to be made with comfort aids such as teddies, comforting smells, soothing music and other helpful reminders that they are safe now and that this is just the mind checking and processing the past.

The child may need help with going to sleep and staying asleep; in addition to the environment and the sensory comforts, other helpful aids include short-term use of melatonin or the equivalent that the doctor can give for a difficult period of time.

## Flashbacks leading to avoidance, anxiety or phobias

We would recognize that if someone was in a car crash, they may take a while getting back into a car and may be more sensitive to the sound of tyres braking fast or the jolts that can happen in a normal car journey. There is little shame regarding this normal reaction. When someone has been hurt or abused at a party or in school, they may try and avoid such settings or seem anxious or phobic, and often be unable to explain why. If they do manage to be physically present, they may look blank, confused, disorientated or scared, but not have the ability to rationally articulate what they feel and why.

## Where do I find help for this area?

The professional who can support the child processing trauma memories is usually trained specifically to do so. The often-suggested modality of CBT (cognitive behavioural therapy) or verbal therapy is generally not fully effective with children who have complex trauma symptoms such as those described in this chapter. This is because the traumatized child can rarely find words to explain what is going on and the parts of the brain needed for CBT are usually not easily accessible due to the stress they feel. The trauma recovery focused lens for dissociative symptoms is not specifically on a qualifying course that I am aware of, and as such the requirements of a psychologist or psychotherapist would be one who has evidence of doing at least an additional week or more of training and has evidence of walking many children through trauma recovery first-hand. If this professional has only helped their own children or only one or two children through to recovery, I would not see that as enough to be appropriate if the child who is needing the help has experienced significant trauma. That level of experience would be sufficient to help facilitate recovery for a child who has experienced Type I trauma but not a child with a more complex, multi-layered traumatic history. Creative psychotherapists would be my preference because of their ability to use creative methods to begin to help process and express subconscious and unconscious emotions, memories and turmoil before words are used.

## Conclusion

This area is the most complex and the most important for complex trauma. There are no short cuts, even though we all wish there were. There are no pills, no medication, no diagnosis that can 'fix this'; instead, the only route is a courageous journey of acknowledging the trauma experience or the trauma of the unmet needs, reducing the shame of this and acknowledging the defence mechanisms and coping strategies that have become automatic, so that the trauma can be eventually processed.

## Resources

A useul therapeutic story book for helping a child who may be dissociative to explore how they feel in a relaxed and not shaming way: *Alex and the Scary Things* by Melissa Moses (2015). Jessica Kingsley Publishers.

My book on dissociation: *The Simple Guide to Complex Trauma and Dissociation* (2020). Jessica Kingsley Publishers.

## Questions to reflect on
### For parents/carers/therapeutic mentors

- What behaviours have you noticed in the child who is distressed that seem to come 'out of nowhere'?

THE SUBCONSCIOUS AND UNCONSCIOUS

- Has the child found CBT or verbal therapy unhelpful and has it increased their shame?
- Does the child often seem to be in denial of what happened?
- What symptoms of dissociation have you noticed?
- How is the child's sleep?
- Do they have flashbacks and what do they do to manage those?
- Who do you know who is qualified and experienced to help process the unconscious memories?

## For therapists

- What place on the Dissociative Continuum do you feel confident to work within?
- Are you familiar with the VIP or the daisy theory and how have you found it helpful? Further training is available based on my book *The Simple Guide to Complex Trauma and Dissociation* (www. traumarecoveryglobal.com).
- Consult my chapter called 'Symptomatology in Complex Trauma and Dissociation (pre-school, early childhood, and school years)' in a book called *The Handbook for Child Complex Trauma and Dissociation: Theory, Research, and Clinical Applications* by Ana Gomez and Jill Hosey (2025).

# CHAPTER 14

# The Mind

Trauma impacts the thinking of a child as well as their body, their unconscious and their emotions, and this can lead to further symptoms of distress as they try and cope with and manage what can be whirling in their head. Van der Kolk (2014) says that 'trauma results in a fundamental reorganization of the way mind and brain manage perceptions. It changes not only how we think and what we think about, but also our very capacity to think' (p.21).

The negative thoughts can start off as thoughts that can be present due a specific experience, but they can grow in quantity and strength, and feel like weeds that take over the 'garden' of the child's mind. It's important that children feel able to describe their thoughts, the worries they have and the power that those seem to have, so that they feel less frightened by what is happening and more able to take control of their thinking. Many children start to worry and then worry about worrying, and things can escalate quickly. Children can hear adults speaking about 'the mental health crisis' and assume that if they have a few negative thoughts, they may be 'broken' or 'have a disorder' or be 'mentally unwell'. These negative thoughts can quickly increase and feel as if they can't be controlled, and then the child feels increasingly powerless, which causes them to panic more and so their thoughts get more intense. This spiral of negative thinking can be worrying to notice, but there are things that adults can do to help stop the escalation of anxious or negative thinking.

## Belonging

Some negative thinking can arise due to feelings that the child doesn't belong and is not liked, and therefore they withdraw and become isolated.

The brain is continually scanning the social environment for signals that tell you if you do or don't belong. When a person gets the signals – many of which are subconscious – that they belong, their stress response systems quiet down, telling them they're safe. They feel regulated and rewarded. But when they get cues that they don't belong, their stress response systems are activated. (Perry & Winfrey, 2021, p.263)

A child may have friends on social media or seem popular, but if they lack the ability to sit down and chat to someone about life and how they feel, they can feel isolated and alone, and begin to wonder why, which can lead to negative thinking about themselves and the world. 'Disconnection is often equated with social rejection, social exclusion, and/or social isolation and these feelings of disconnection actually share the same neural pathways with feelings of physical pain. It can hurt as much as physical pain' (Brown, 2021, p.171). We need to create space for children to chat about their friendships so that we can help them navigate through some of the complexities and feel that they have connection and belonging and are known, seen and appreciated by peers.

'I never did feel like I belonged because I was just in my own world. I was described as a loner but what could I do? No one could come too near me because I had too many secrets. I had to just survive.' *Liz, aged 18*

## Triggers

Triggers are the sudden invasive thoughts or reactions to something that the child sees, smells, feels or touches that causes them to relive the traumatic experience. It can cause a fast reaction as if they were back in the original trauma, and others around them may be confused due to the behaviour seeming to be so out of context. For example, someone may have been abused by a person who smells of smoke; the child walks into a room, smells smoke and runs out of the room screaming as if they are dying. They may soon afterwards feel embarrassed and awkward as they know that the room they walked into was a safe and friendly family home and the smoke was just a log fire, which they love.

Alternatively, the child may be doing a maths test and be confident until they get towards the end, when they may panic as they realize that they may not do as well as they had hoped; immediately, they have thoughts of being useless and stupid, which causes them to feel shame, and that makes them feel that they are not safe and so they shout, scream, kick or run. The child can then dread tests because they can feel the impending sense of failure and shame, which causes them to feel as if they are being abused even when the teacher setting the test is being kind and gentle. The cycle of impending shame leading to avoidance or anger can be easy to spot when you understand what triggers can look like and can see how children can feel powerless in a behaviour cycle that they don't understand. The child can learn to explore the triggers as they slowly process the trauma memories; the sensory triggers become clear and lose the shock that causes the instinctive reactions that can create shame and confusion.

## Eight basic techniques to help bring calm

Here are some ways to help children who start to show signs of negative thinking:

- Acknowledge it and don't brush it away. Don't tell them not to worry or minimize their distress, because that causes them to disconnect from you or to avoid telling you what's going on.
- Show empathy for them, even if the worry or thoughts seem unlikely to be a real threat or justified worry. Try and stand in their shoes and remember being their age, and show kindness and empathy for them as they explain to you some of what is going on in their mind.
- Help them to write or draw their thoughts or worries, so that they can see them. This way of 'capturing' thoughts is a powerful way to reduce their impact and enables them to feel clearer and less whirly.
- Spend some time chatting to them about their thoughts or worries and what they could do to reduce any stress or anxiety in practical ways first. If there is nothing practical to do (for example, sourcing a new pack of pens for school so they won't get into trouble, or helping them find their lost football boots or writing an email to a teacher to explain why they couldn't do

something), then work out what is the worst scenario so that they can hopefully see that it is not as bad as their mind led them to believe.

- Teach them to do some different calming techniques or suggest they write a journal of their thoughts and what they think about those thoughts.
- Provide sensory activities that bring a sense of calm to their body and nervous system, such as holding and stroking a favourite soft toy or cushion, smelling some hand cream or a candle, listening to some calming music or drinking a warm comforting drink.
- Do some breathing exercises with them that help them relax their breath and lose the tension they feel around their tummy, neck or shoulders.
- Suggest they take up a new hobby that is creative or physical and helps them grow in skill. Although learning a new skill can be tough at the start, it can bring great comfort and confidence. Both creative and physical activities are good for the brain, nervous system and health of the child, and are far better than screen time or being bored.

## Breathing exercises

A child can be shown how to slow down their breathing when they feel stressed, angry or scared, and they can grasp that this change in rhythm of breathing can help them move from their sympathetic nervous system state (fight and flight) to their parasympathetic nervous system (rest and digest). Their heart rate slows down and they can begin to feel calm. Ironically, some children can find paying attention to their breathing difficult or even triggering, especially if their trauma has caused them to gasp, cough or struggle to breathe. Other children may find such exercises helpful for them to feel calmer and more relaxed when their thoughts are racing and they are beginning to panic and dysregulate. Here are some simple techniques:

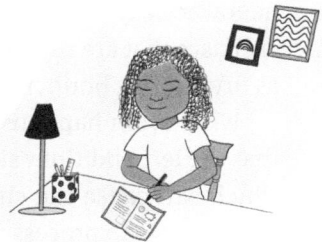

- Hand breathing – trace your hand outline while breathing through your nose and out through your mouth. Up the thumb breathing in, and breathing out as your finger traces back down the thumb, breathing in through your nose as your finger traces up the index finger and then out through your mouth as you come down the other side of the finger and so on. This needs to be at the pace that is relaxing and not stressful.
- Blowing bubbles or blowing table tennis balls across the floor.
- Stretching up 'to the sky' while breathing in and then, after a count of three, releasing the breath dramatically like a balloon losing its air and flopping. Wait and feel the sensation on the body, which should be slightly tingly, buzzy or calming.

## Physical calming techniques to use with negative thoughts

There are lots of other easy-to-learn techniques that help the mind stop whirling so much because they redirect the thoughts and attention to something else.

Alongside breathing games and exercises that the children can learn, there are some other movements that intentionally help a child to feel less out of control, less stressed and more able to think clearly. Bilateral stimulation is the back-and-forth (often left to right, sometimes diagonal) movement across the body's midline that promotes neural activity (Laliotis et al., 2021). There are some bilateral stimulating exercises that are rhythmic and can help reduce stress for all ages, such as drumming, bouncing balls to each other and clapping games.

What often happens when we are stressed or feel overwhelmed is that the left and right sides of the brain don't communicate very well, which can cause the child to feel stuck, be reactive, have flashbacks and struggle to process what worries them, their trauma or their shock. Our right brain holds the emotions and sensory memories, and our left brain holds the narrative and thoughts, and when they are integrated, there is less confusion and stress. The overwhelming feelings of distress can be decreased with these exercises, and the relationship between the two sides of the brain can grow in strength, which enables more emotional regulation and easier access to words which describe feelings. They can be used to say a positive affirmation where the fear thoughts were filling their minds, such as 'I am able to do this difficult thing', while they do the exercises. Bilateral stimulation simultaneously engages both sides of the body or brain in a way that activates the brain's natural healing processes. It can help the child relax, regulate their emotion and integrate their experiences.

Here are some helpful bilateral stimulating exercises:

- *The butterfly hug:* This is a simple way of crossing our arms across our body and patting ourselves. It may sound daft, but it is a helpful way of comforting and grounding, and also offers some bilateral stimulation which helps the person to process their thinking and feel better.
- *Rhythmic clapping games:* These can be mirrored or copied by an adult from a child or vice versa. This can work well in a pair or in a group and can help the child to feel connected and not alone, but also helps the right and left sides of the brain to connect, which brings a sense of calm.
- *Marching or drumming:* This can help stimulate the two sides of the brain and also bring a sense of fun and order as you try and drum or march in rhythm with the other person. This can lead to laughter but also all bilateral stimulation can bring a sense of calm.
- *Strong sitting:* This is a way of crossing over many parts of the body that aims to cross over the brain too, so that the overwhelm begins to decrease. You cross over your arms by putting your arms out in front of you and putting the back of the hands together and then crossing them over and pulling in the arms towards the tummy to hold by your neck. If you do this while sitting crossed-legged too, it's a great way to then move into some breathing exercises.
- *Rocking in a hammock:* This can be helpful when there is a sense of rhythm. It can also recreate or heal early experiences of being a baby where the child may or should have been rocked rhyth-mically in a soothing way.
- *Walking, running or cycling:* These activities use the two sides of the body in rhythm and can have a similar impact.

## Therapeutic story books and psychoeducation books

These can be incredibly useful to help children of all ages feel less afraid of what is happening to them, which can de-escalate their anxiety or stress.

The story books tell stories of animals or children who struggle with different challenges such as anxiety, worry or overwhelm. They explain what it feels like for them and what they do to feel better. Psychoeducation books help explain important concepts of how humans feel about things, and this decreases shame and increases a sense of normality. Many children have a sense of relief and learn faster through these books than through the adult trying to explain it because it is less intense and again stimulates both sides of the brain.

Some ideas for therapeutic books for worry, anxiety and thinking challenges are:

- *Charley Chatty and the Wiggly Worry Worm: A story about insecurity and attention-seeking* by Sarah Naish and Rosie Jefferies (2016). Jessica Kingsley Publishers.
- *Binnie the Baboon Anxiety and Stress Activity Book: A Therapeutic Story with Creative and CBT Activities to Help Children Aged 5–10 Who Worry* by Karen Treisman (2019). Jessica Kingsley Publishers.
- *Help! I've Got an Alarm Bell Going Off in My Head!* by K.L Aspden (2015). Jessica Kingsley Publishers.
- *Starving the Anxiety Gremlin for Children Aged 5–9: A Cognitive Behavioural Therapy Workbook on Anxiety Management* by Kate Collins-Donnelly (2014). Jessica Kingsley Publishers.
- *Creative Ways to Help Children Manage Anxiety: Ideas and Activities for Working Therapeutically with Worried Children and Their Families* by Fiona Zandt and Suzanne Barrett (2020). Jessica Kingsley Publishers.
- *William Wobbly and the Very Bad Day: A Story About When Feelings Become Too Big* by Sarah Naish and Rosie Jefferies (2016). Jessica Kingsley Publishers.
- *A Terrible Thing Happened: A Story for Children Who Have Witnessed Violence or Trauma* by Margaret Holmes (2000). Magination Press.

## The Safe Place visualization

This is a simple exercise to do with a child, where they spend time creating their ideal, safe place. They need to be helped to think about their favourite kind of space, what it looks like, what it sounds and smells like and who would be invited there. They can be invited to draw it, make it from clay or construct a tent with blankets or cardboard, and to spend time reflecting on what it feels like to be in it. The aim is that eventually they can hold the memory of the space in their mind, and then when they feel distressed or dysregulated, they are able to go there in their mind and feel the relaxation and relief of being somewhere that feels safe.

This exercise isn't just a comforting way to imagine a lovely place; it is a way to activate the parasympathetic nervous system (rest and digest) out of the sympathetic nervous system (fight and flight) so that the child can begin to think, reflect and feel calm again. This is helpful for children who have experienced Type I trauma but can be used with children who have experienced Type II or III trauma. It may also fuel derealization, so it's important to notice how long the child is in that space.

## Overthinking and catastrophizing

Children can begin to panic about their worries and find themselves stuck in overthinking where they increasingly seem to sink into hopelessness or panic. This is when it is important to introduce different methods for them to externalize what is going on, because when it stays internalized, it grows bigger than it really is when it comes 'into the light of day'.

Catastrophizing can begin to grow when a child is exposed to stories of disaster that panic them and make them feel as if the same may happen to them. They can then find themselves preparing for such an event and overthinking what could happen, and then this can escalate into panic when the slightest hint of a disaster occurs. For example, as an adult you may exclaim that you may run out of petrol if you don't find a petrol station, and they disproportionately panic that they will be stuck in a car, in the middle of nowhere and starve to death and be found as dead bodies in a year. This kind of thinking often happens due to exposure to films, media and books which they have not been able to contextualize effectively and have fed an increase in anxiety and panic. The child can need reassurance from adults where they explain what measures are in place to stay safe and avoid disasters, until the child no longer panics in different settings.

## Self-hatred, self-blame, self-doubt and self-loathing

A traumatized child can struggle with self-hatred or self-loathing due to what they have endured. Research suggests that those who experienced interpersonal trauma, especially violence and sexual abuse can be most impacted (Hyland *et al.*, 2017; Gilbert, 2015; Weindl & Lueger-Schuster, 2018). Survivors of trauma can blame themselves for what happened and view themselves as deserving to what happened to them. These painful thought patterns can create a crippling sense of turmoil and cause a lack of confidence in connecting with others, which leads to increased isolation, which then leads to increased self-hatred, blame, doubt and loathing. The irony of these spirals is that they usually begin in the context of being a part of a friendship of some kind, but they creep in as gnawing fear which then escalates and begins to stop the connection completely. The small doubts or painful feelings of shame are not able to be resolved in the relationship and so seem to eat away at them, causing growing insecurities and turmoil that usually remain internalized and therefore unable to be challenged, until they have grown to take up so much space in the child's mind internally that it's hard for them to listen to anyone.

This is especially the struggle for teenagers, and it is important to notice immediately if there is any self-doubt or self-hatred and to quickly but gently bring reassurance that all humans are different, that there is no perfection for anyone in any area and that being kind to others is a far higher value to focus on. During puberty, the child can feel fraught with insecurity about the way they look and how others perceive them, and grow in terror of rejection, not fitting in, not being accepted by those whose opinions they care about. It's almost impossible to walk straight through puberty with total confidence and no insecurity or self-doubt.

Social media has not been kind to a generation who are now exposed to opinions about what we 'should' look like in every area of our body and what we should think about everything and who is 'right' and who is 'wrong'. This changes faster than anyone can keep up with, leaving it a high possibility that if a young person looks and listens from a place of fear and insecurity without any trusted older voice of comfort, reassurance and calm, they could easily panic and become distressed. They need us as adults to point out people we admire and why we admire them for their kindness, generosity and building others up, and explain how we don't admire people who have wealth or popularity if they are not kind. This needs to be regularly reflected on as we watch TV or scroll through social media so that the young people grow up less likely to believe the lie of what is presented as ultimate success.

## Fantasy and struggling with reality

Some children end up becoming addicted to gaming and can struggle to engage with others outside this setting. Their reality becomes distorted, and the day-to-day tasks of life seem to be dull and meaningless compared to the colours, graphics, sounds, power and excitement of the dopamine-releasing games that hook the player to increased time in a fantasy world. For children affected by poverty, trauma, loss, pain and turmoil, this other world can offer hope and interest in an otherwise dull and disappointing world where they can struggle to have a sense of purpose and hope for their future. While gaming can bring some connection with others and some positive winning experiences, it can also overwhelm the child, especially pre-puberty, and this overwhelm can be damaging to their ability to find satisfaction in simpler enjoyments such as reading, sports and exploring an outside area. For some children, it is a way to escape the pain and can develop into dissociation, which is a coping mechanism that exists on a continuum. For short-term relief, or connection when physical connection is challenging, or when distraction is essential for a child's wellbeing, or when isolation or turmoil is too overwhelming, gaming can be a helpful aid. However, it needs to be monitored by ensuring that other activities can be as rewarding as the gaming, and the reality of life can be differentiated from the fantasy of the online world.

## Depression, sadness, withdrawal

Some children can find things too much, and the sadness that they may carry from a traumatic event of some kind may grow in size rather than shrink as it changes their worldview. Sometimes, trauma can be like putting on a pair of glasses that are dark and wondering why others don't seem to see the darkness but can laugh and jump and run and giggle. It can feel confusing for the child watching on and feeling as if they are in a different reality.

Sadness is an entirely normal and natural reaction to experiencing difficult things or to a traumatic experience. Some people describe sadness as coming and going in waves, but where they can still enjoy some aspects of life and still look forward to things in the future. Depression is different and more intense. Sometimes, it can be hard to distinguish between sadness and depression, but usually people who struggle with depression have more of a constant feeling of sadness that rarely seems to go and is impacting every area of their life. They now don't even enjoy the things they used to look forward to and they feel stuck and hopeless. This sadness stops them being with others, which makes it worse, and they begin to lose hope that things can change. The child needs to find help by this stage.

There are signs to look out for. You need to take action to stop it getting worse when the child:

- stops enjoying activities they used to enjoy
- is not getting enough exercise, fresh air, sleep or food
- wants to stay in bed all the time or seems to lie about things
- struggles to talk to friends or relatives who they used to enjoy being with
- is beginning to self-harm or speak negatively about themselves.

## Anxiety and worry

Sometimes anxiety can be a feeling that happens when a child has an event or an experience that they are worried about. They also may have worries that grow in both intensity and duration, especially when there doesn't seem to be enough choice, comfort or support. It is important to differentiate between normal worries that most children have about changes, challenges or circumstances and anxiety that seems to impact their whole life and limits what they can do.

Sometimes anxiety can sound more like specific worries such as

'I hate myself' or 'I hate you' or 'I am probably going to mess this up' or 'I am not going to that club anymore as I am rubbish'. These sentences often show the fear about being rejected, failure, loneliness or overwhelm. They may want to avoid school because they are worried about exams, tests, friendships or being shamed. Some children are more sensitive to environments that are busy and purpose-driven, and they can become anxious in the speed of the day. They also may express that they have tummy aches or headaches or have trouble sleeping. They need consistent co-regulation, emotional connection, kindness, reassurance and suggestions for how to do what they need to do without anxiety taking control of their life. They need empathy and encouragement in equal measure, and the adult needs to be attuned to how far to encourage them to do things that are difficult or whether they need help to avoid them because they will cause too much stress. It's not easy to get this balance right, but it is important to speak to professionals who have experience in this and are able to help before things escalate quickly. When a child's worry continues past one specific event, it is important to quickly de-escalate and stop the child feeling stuck in cycles that they can really struggle to break. The earlier they can have help, the easier it is to help them carry on with normal life with fewer interruptions.

Simple ways to de-escalate anxiety:

- All the activities previously listed in this chapter.
- The 333-grounding game where they have to spot three things that begin with, say, the letter C: one that they hear, one that they can see, one that they can feel. They can move on to another letter as they become distracted and their prefrontal cortex begins to experience more neural energy so that they can now think and reflect a bit more.
- The ABC game where you take turns having to think of an animal/plant/person who starts with that letter of the alphabet.
- Safe places that enable them to feel calm and sensorily comfortable.
- Music playlists that have been created to help them calm and breathe easily.

## Suicidal thinking or suicidal ideation

Sadly, sometimes a child can grow in feelings of turmoil and distress that can lead them to feel increasingly hopeless, and they can begin to want the distress to end. Fisher (2017) describes the experience of being traumatized:

> feeling helpless, overwhelmed, inadequate, vulnerable, terrified, and alone, the lived experience is that there is nowhere to turn, nowhere to hide, no one to help. The only resources upon which each individual can draw reside in the body; disconnection, numbing, dissociation, neurochemicals such as adrenaline and endorphins, and the animal survival responses of fight, flight, freeze, submit, and attach for survival. These are desperate times requiring desperate measures. (p.126)

Most young people who speak about what it was like to feel suicidal say this very important sentence: *I didn't want to die but I wanted the pain to stop.*

This is always important to remember because while they know that after the turmoil has begun to decrease, they can lose sight of it when they are in the height of big, overwhelming feelings that seem suffocating and too much to cope with. They are sometimes needing attention – but that's not the same as attention seeking, which is made to sound as if they should 'grow up' and stop being so demanding. Attention is a need for children to become healthy and for adults to stay healthy, and when a child has struggled to have consistent emotional connection with an adult or when a young person has struggled to have that adult attachment and not had enough of the positive, emotionally accepting and connecting peer relationships, they can need some attention. It is often said that the children who ask for attention sometimes ask in the most unloving of ways, which is not because they are 'broken' or 'stupid' but because they are desperate. We need to acknowledge that and build some bridges, follow their lead and try and help them feel safer, cared for, validated, known, seen, heard and accepted. These positive feelings of connection can decrease a lot of the feelings of life being 'too much' and therefore can decrease the feeling that suicide is the only available option to stop the pain.

## Using the Betsy VIP model to help

A tried and tested method that I have found to work well with children who are suicidal is when I have spent time using the daisy theory (TRFM® Tool 9) and especially the VIP (TRFM® Tool 8). It can be easy to draw the three circles and talk about how the professional part of them may actually still want to become an actor/photographer/doctor/pilot/writer and so on, but the inner-child part is stuck with fear of failure and that they can't do anything they want to because the vulnerable part of them hates life and is stuck in pain. When they can see that the whole of them doesn't want to die, but only one part does, they can find a little bit more strength to keep going. It refocuses their thinking to see it's just one part of them taking up too much power, which isn't fair on the whole of them.

This can work well, but only in the context of an adult having built a therapeutic or supportive relationship with them before the crisis or by introducing the concept to them in the moment of a crisis with confidence that we are *not* minimizing the level of turmoil and pain and distress. We use it to wonder if there is one tiny part of them that still maybe wants to…see a sunset/dance with a lover/make a beautiful piece of art/giggle until they can hardly breathe/see that city/breathe the sea air again. Using tools like this is so much about the way we speak, the body language we present with, the tone of voice, the facial expression, and our ability to perceive what is going on with the child and what 'way in' can we use to bring a ray of hope and then grow that hope until stability is established.

## A safety plan

It is vital for the child to have access to a safety plan, to help them de-escalate if they begin to feel unstable. It can be as simple as this:

**A crisis plan template to create with your young person when they are feeling calm, to be ready for when they have a low period/crisis or suicidal thoughts**

What can I do right now to distract or comfort me?

. . . . . . . . . . . . . . . . . . . . . . . . . . . . . . . . . . . . . . . . . . . . . . . . . . . . . . . . . . . . .

. . . . . . . . . . . . . . . . . . . . . . . . . . . . . . . . . . . . . . . . . . . . . . . . . . . . . . . . . . . . .

. . . . . . . . . . . . . . . . . . . . . . . . . . . . . . . . . . . . . . . . . . . . . . . . . . . . . . . . . . . . .

. . . . . . . . . . . . . . . . . . . . . . . . . . . . . . . . . . . . . . . . . . . . . . . . . . . . . . . . . . . . .

What could I do to focus on something positive or fun?

. . . . . . . . . . . . . . . . . . . . . . . . . . . . . . . . . . . . . . . . . . . . . . . . . . . . . . . . . . . . .

. . . . . . . . . . . . . . . . . . . . . . . . . . . . . . . . . . . . . . . . . . . . . . . . . . . . . . . . . . . . .

. . . . . . . . . . . . . . . . . . . . . . . . . . . . . . . . . . . . . . . . . . . . . . . . . . . . . . . . . . . . .

. . . . . . . . . . . . . . . . . . . . . . . . . . . . . . . . . . . . . . . . . . . . . . . . . . . . . . . . . . . . .

Is there something that would make me safer?

. . . . . . . . . . . . . . . . . . . . . . . . . . . . . . . . . . . . . . . . . . . . . . . . . . . . . . . . . . . . .

. . . . . . . . . . . . . . . . . . . . . . . . . . . . . . . . . . . . . . . . . . . . . . . . . . . . . . . . . . . . .

. . . . . . . . . . . . . . . . . . . . . . . . . . . . . . . . . . . . . . . . . . . . . . . . . . . . . . . . . . . . .

. . . . . . . . . . . . . . . . . . . . . . . . . . . . . . . . . . . . . . . . . . . . . . . . . . . . . . . . . . . . .

Who can I contact to support me?

. . . . . . . . . . . . . . . . . . . . . . . . . . . . . . . . . . . . . . . . . . . . . . . . . . . . . . . . . . . . .

. . . . . . . . . . . . . . . . . . . . . . . . . . . . . . . . . . . . . . . . . . . . . . . . . . . . . . . . . . . . .

. . . . . . . . . . . . . . . . . . . . . . . . . . . . . . . . . . . . . . . . . . . . . . . . . . . . . . . . . . . . .

. . . . . . . . . . . . . . . . . . . . . . . . . . . . . . . . . . . . . . . . . . . . . . . . . . . . . . . . . . . . .

Which professional can I contact?

. . . . . . . . . . . . . . . . . . . . . . . . . . . . . . . . . . . . . . . . . . . . . . . . . . . . . . . .

. . . . . . . . . . . . . . . . . . . . . . . . . . . . . . . . . . . . . . . . . . . . . . . . . . . . . . . .

. . . . . . . . . . . . . . . . . . . . . . . . . . . . . . . . . . . . . . . . . . . . . . . . . . . . . . . .

. . . . . . . . . . . . . . . . . . . . . . . . . . . . . . . . . . . . . . . . . . . . . . . . . . . . . . . .

Emergency numbers for professionals:

. . . . . . . . . . . . . . . . . . . . . . . . . . . . . . . . . . . . . . . . . . . . . . . . . . . . . . . .

. . . . . . . . . . . . . . . . . . . . . . . . . . . . . . . . . . . . . . . . . . . . . . . . . . . . . . . .

. . . . . . . . . . . . . . . . . . . . . . . . . . . . . . . . . . . . . . . . . . . . . . . . . . . . . . . .

. . . . . . . . . . . . . . . . . . . . . . . . . . . . . . . . . . . . . . . . . . . . . . . . . . . . . . . .

(de Thierry, 2020, pp.134–135)

## Conclusion

When a child's mind begins to be plagued with hopeless thoughts that are escalating, it can be frightening for an adult to know what to do to bring hope and help. The earlier the negative thoughts are seen to be present, the easier it is to de-escalate the child's anxiety, depression or distress with confident help and to enable them to externalize their thinking that seems to be 'catching' and 'multiplying'. However, at any period, our brains are malleable and flexible, and we can see change by externalizing, noticing, acknowledging, validating and offering alternative methods to find calm, hope and pleasure again. The most important thing to remember is that the child who is distressed is desperate to escape the pain and we need to help them with suggestions and ideas until some of them 'click' and seem to work for them. We can't give up hope, and when we feel that we cannot continue, we need to find support ourselves so that we can keep going.

## Questions to reflect on
### For parents/carers/therapeutic mentors

- Out of the eight basic techniques to bring calm, which ones have worked for you or the child you are supporting?
- Which physical calming techniques or breathing exercises have you found work best or do you want to try out?
- Have you tried using therapeutic story books or psychoeducation books to help the child understand themselves better?
- Which areas are the biggest challenge right now – overthinking, catastrophizing, self-hatred, self-blame, self-doubt or self-loathing – and what could you do to help reduce them?
- Does the child currently struggle with sadness, depression or suicidal thinking? What could you do to help them?
- Have you made a safety plan for a child who seems to be unstable, so that they know what to do if they quickly decrease in stability and safety?

### For therapists

- What tools have you used and found to work with children with challenges in their thinking, self-concept or suicidality? Which ones could you try?
- In which areas would you say you are growing in confidence and skill, and in which areas would you say that you feel very confident?

# CHAPTER 15

# Relationships

When a child experiences trauma, it is usually in the context of relationships. They were either traumatized because a person hurt them intentionally or as a mistake, or they were hurt because an adult wasn't there to stop them being hurt. Therefore, trauma impacts the child's relationships and understanding of how relationships work, and the younger they were to experience trauma, the more they are negatively impacted in this area. Chapter 3 explores how to build positive relationships with the child, and so this chapter is an exploration of some of the additional issues that may arise.

## Trust issues

It makes sense that a child may not find it easy to trust an adult, even when the adult reassures them that they are trustworthy. Trusting others comes from the repetitive positive experience of trusting, which has felt comfortable and pleasurable. If a child has trusted an adult who has then violated that trust, it leaves them with an internal conflict where they subconsciously recognize their need for adults to protect them, but they know that some adults can harm them. This causes a lot of children to be tentative in trusting an adult, or they withdraw, hide, watch them from a distance or test them with difficult situations to see how they react. Children test us in many ways, to see if we are trustworthy, and the relationship can grow in strength when we react in ways that don't shock, scare or overwhelm them. Music (2019) suggests that 'good relationships, including good psychotherapists, are characterized not by harmony, but by continuous disruption and repair' (p.35).

## Trust issues with their peers

Children who have experienced trauma can be confused about relationships and can be clingy or controlling or anxious, especially about if they are still liked, loved and included. Sometimes they can seem to be unbothered and relaxed about if they belong. Both these reactions demonstrate the underlying fear of being rejected, abandoned, hurt, mocked, exposed or violated. It can take time for them to build trust with others, and this can be frustrating as the child may 'test' the loyalty and trustworthiness over time.

## Betrayal

With interpersonal trauma, which is usually Type II or III trauma, the impact is one where the child feels betrayed by the person who should be caring for and protecting them. Even when it doesn't seem logical to us as adults, the child is aware of how powerless they are without adults to help them, and therefore when the help isn't there or when the person who should be helping hurts them instead, they feel shocked, betrayed and deeply hurt. Betrayal trauma is the child feeling violated because they had placed trust in that adult who has used that trust to harm them. It can be the deepest sense of rejection, shock and turmoil as they try and make sense of what has happened, and therefore it usually causes the symptoms that would signify complex trauma. Often, the adult who has betrayed the child continues to be present and so the child must adjust to protecting and defending themselves. Research asserts that traumas that are perpetrated by trusted individuals or within the family are more psychologically harmful than other trauma types (Gamache Martin, Van Ryzin & Dishion, 2016). This is explained further in *The Simple Guide to Attachment Difficulties* (de Thierry, 2019) and *The Simple Guide to Complex Trauma and Dissociation* (de Thierry, 2020). The child could have formed an attachment subconscious template that is called disorganized attachment. This usually causes dissociation to form in order to help the child stay alive but not feel the shock and turmoil in their day-to-day interactions.

Children who have been abused, psychologically, physically or sexually, can grow up subconsciously expecting more pain and turmoil. It can feel 'normal' to be hurt and harmed by another person because they have not experienced the feeling of being defended or protected. This can then lead to the child not speaking about it if they are hurt again by someone, because they think that will happen all of their life. It can also cause them to feel 'safer' when things are dangerous than when things are calm and happy, because it feels 'normal'.

## People pleasing

Traumatized children become painfully aware of the power that adults have over them and so they can develop a terror of experiencing further harm from them. The most recognized responses to threat are the fight, flight or freeze responses, but they could also react in other instinctive ways to stay alive in the face of danger. The fawn response is an automatic reaction when fighting or fleeing would be a greater risk to their sense of safety. The fawn response can feel activating in the face of disempowerment as the child intentionally offers help, support and people-pleasing behaviours, which can bring a de-escalation in the instance. This type of response can also help the child to avoid being the target of anger and aggression by being helpful towards the adult who poses a threat. The behaviour can simultaneously bring a sense of calm, regulate the adult's behaviour and emotions and protect the child from being the focus of any negative emotional expression (Schlote, 2023).

The fear of adult emotions and reactions can cause the child to avoid adults' attention or to work hard to please them in order to avoid any anger, disappointment or frustration and what could happen if they sparked off any of these negative emotions in the adult. They can become habitual in their avoidance of relationships or avoidance of anything that may provoke anger, and this can fuel a desire to please everyone around them. This can continue into adulthood and impact all relationships and career choices, so it's important to help them explore this when they are adolescents or young adults. When a child is compliant with their primary caregivers, they are usually less able to assert their own opinion or choice regarding other matters and can find it harder to say 'no' to adults or peers who want to hurt them. They may shrug their shoulders and be avoidant of making decisions in case they 'get told off' or have adults angry with them. A healthy child is able to discuss decisions with their parents in a way that is reasonable and rational, where they expect to be seen, heard and their opinion valued, if not always adhered to.

## Over-dependency and attachment anxiety

Sometimes, however, children can become frightened of losing the adult who seems to be trustworthy. They can become anxious about leaving them or they need to control them and how they spend their time, so that they feel less powerless. The child can refuse to go to different settings or complete work that they are asked to do without the chosen adult being present. I have written at length about attachment challenges and what to do with children who have experienced attachment trauma in *The Simple Guide to Attachment Difficulties* (2019).

When a parent or carer is too relaxed and isn't able to hold firm boundaries, the child can feel that they are not safe because the adult feels more like a peer and no one seems to be the grown-up.

Alternatively, when a parent or carer is too authoritarian or controlling or dominant, the child isn't able to express themselves or their feelings and so is left unvalidated and not feeling understood, with unexpressed emotion.

## Rupture and repair

When something goes wrong in a relationship, it can be an opportunity for repair, and, after rupture, the repair can be healing if it is navigated with that intention. For children who have experienced loss, rejection or abandonment, it may cause instant terror if the adult isn't emotionally available, kind, attuned or reassuring. However, if the adult then says sorry and explains why they weren't their normal self, then while the child may struggle with that, they also may be able to slowly grasp that humans can try their best but sometimes do mess up, and that they can also repair the relationship. This can eventually enable the child's understanding of relationships to grow in strength and confidence and cause less anxiety.

Ruptures can be of two main subtypes: withdrawal and confrontation (Safran & Muran, 2000). The child can withdraw from the adult and disengage. They may use long silences, minimal responses, changing the subject of the conversation, or abstract intellectual talk. Or the child may move towards the adult by 'readily complying', at the cost of denying their own needs. In confrontational ruptures, the child may be angry and express frustration with the adult helping them. Offering therapeutic care and kindness, where ruptures can be worked through and repaired, can strengthen the child's trust in adults and give them hope and tools to be able to know that rupture and repair are tolerable and not impossible.

## Lying

They may be secretive about things in their life that they feel shame about, or are confused or embarrassed about. They may find their life dull and boring and lie to make them sound more interesting so that they can feel connected, or they could lie because of their derealization, where they may confuse reality with fantasy and be unsure of what the truth actually is. The more positive relationships the child has, the less likely they are to need to lie, but when they do lie, it is important to know that there are usually good reasons, so telling them to stop lying is counterproductive. Lying is a defence mechanism to try and help them feel less vulnerable to being further hurt by people around them. The only long-term, healthy way to decrease lying is simply to increase emotional safety. Sometimes a child lies because they have not seen the value of truth and not seen that modelled. Perry and Szalavitz (2010) explore a child who lied to everyone and the reasons behind it with the reflection that 'in his family, there was little trust and, therefore, little motivation to tell the truth unless it could be used to manipulate someone...he was taught that lying was the best way to get what you wanted' (p.101).

Sometimes the child may feel as if they are lying or look guilty as they attempt to speak of something terrifying that has happened. This could be due to the lies that adults have said to the child, such as 'No one will believe you' and 'Everyone knows you are a liar', which cause them to doubt their own memories and experience. They can wonder if

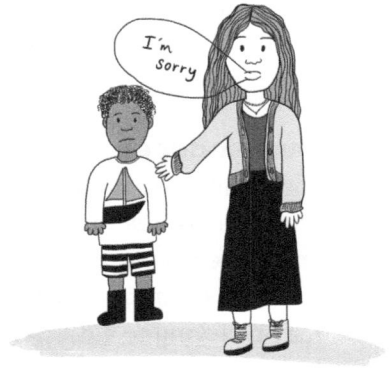

it is true and almost hope it isn't as they hear their own voice speaking of the unspeakable.

'I was called a liar by my dad all the time. Even when my boyfriend met him, the first thing he told him about me was that I was a liar. He said nothing positive about me. I mean how was I meant to keep the family secrets of control, manipulation, physical abuse and threats? No one could come to my house as my mum shouted and could do anything violent even if a friend was there, so I had to tell teachers at school that I groaned, sighed and looked blank because my aunt was ill with cancer. What else could I do? I was stuck with them.' *Julia, aged 23, looking back at school life*

## Over-independence

Some children can be viewed as independent and it can sometimes be seen as a positive sign of development. However, if the child is young and there is a history of trauma, they may be acting this way due to feeling insecure about adults and how they are perceived by them. They may be trying to earn the adult's praise and affirmation by being so 'grown up' or responsible. They may have had so many experiences with adults that have rendered them terrified, powerless and overwhelmed that they have decided to ensure that they no longer need any adults to care for them.

## Therapy and therapeutic mentoring

We cannot make anyone work with us, but we recognize that many children who have experienced trauma may well consider spending time with one adult on their own in a small room as a nightmare. What would enable them to trust the adult? The qualifications or the smile? The warm words or the toys? Many children have been hurt by those who were responsible for caring for them and so they would now rather be anywhere other than in such a situation where they feel powerless to an adult's agenda and plan. They will need to slowly build the possibility of trust, over time, in ways where they feel less powerless. Co-creating spaces and plans for the time spent is not a luxury for these children but vital for them to be able to explore safety.

Forcing a child to go to therapy is rarely going to work, but helping them understand more about the therapist, the space that they would be going to, having a visit to see around and feel less powerless about the possibility can be important. At the therapy centres I have founded, we work hard to have interesting toys, activities and creative materials that we know the child may like when they come for a visit. We then get to know the child and make sure that whatever they are interested in, we try and have available to help them build a relationship with us, until they trust us enough not to need that as a distraction. We have used car engines, graffiti painting, cake making, smoothie creating and large constructions to help a child get to know us and start the process of trust and wanting to come to therapy. We certainly don't blame them for needing extra help to begin to trust an adult they don't know, when the reason they need to come for therapy is that they have been hurt by an adult. We have an open-door policy where they can stay connected long term and we work with tools that enable healing in all the areas that the trauma has impacted.

## PACE

The PACE model (Hughes & Golding, 2012, p.14) for building relationships can be very easy to remember and helpful.

**Playfulness:** Always keeping play at the centre of all the interactions where trauma and recovery are the focus.

**Acceptance:** Making sure that we communicate verbally and in our behaviour and emotions and body language that while some things have been difficult, we believe in a better time together and that we, the adult, accept the child. We accept the child as they are and want them to feel that we are not judging them or pitying them.

**Curiosity:** An important element of building a relationship. It is not being nosey but being interested in how the child is known and who they are really are!

**Empathy:** This is vital because we don't really know what it is like to be in their shoes and so we need to imagine and listen so that we can show we care and value them.

## Conclusion

Relationships are central to the experience of being a human. Every adult and child needs to feel that they are part of a group of others who know and care for them. When a child has experienced Type I trauma, they need the reassurance and kindness of adults to help them journey through the process of recovery. They will be less likely to be able to recover without an attentive adult who understands the process and journey. Children who have experienced Type II or III trauma will probably have confusion about their need for adult care, and yet still fear adults. This can result in challenging behaviours that can lead to the child being further misunderstood and even rejected and isolated. Relationships can be life changing when we understand their power to help another person.

## Questions to reflect on
### For parents/carers/therapeutic mentors

- Do you know what attachment style the child has? Are they secure or anxious, ambivalent or disorganized?
- What is their biggest fear in relationships, and their biggest need?
- Have they experienced betrayal trauma?
- Are they clingy or over-independent?
- Have you been able to turn some negative ruptures into stronger repairs?

### For therapists

- Have you studied attachment and disorganized attachment? What attachment styles do you feel able to work with in a recovery-focused way?
- How have you found the theme of betrayal present in the therapy sessions and how have you experienced that?

# CHAPTER 16

# Processing the Trauma Memories

This is the stage that people would ideally like to get on with as soon as possible, and you may even have skipped the few last chapters to be able to learn how to help the child process the traumatic memories so that they can 'get back on track' with their life again.

The reason that I assert with passion that verbal therapy or short-term therapy is not suitable for children who have experienced complex or interpersonal trauma is because to speak about the trauma, which would always be an element of being able to process it, by its very nature can push them beyond the safety of coping mechanisms such as denial or avoidance. The words can be too painful to speak and beyond horrific to hear. The possibility of the listener not leaning in and sensing the profound terror and shock of words that tell snippets of the story of violation, betrayal, abandonment and loss is agonizing. However, there is relief to be found when an adult intuitively senses the moment, the fragility and power of the words, and can represent what should be the response from any human to another who tells of any traumatic experience. They can carry that on their face, their body posture and tone of voice, where warmth, care, genuine empathy and compassion are felt in the room. This can be a moment of profound healing and relief. It can be monumental.

If a child has just experienced a traumatic situation and is able to speak about it, then it is important to enable them to do so safely, and we should not slow them down or make it complicated. In fact, Silberg (2012) says that 'our therapeutic attempts to process traumatic events with children should try to approximate the normalcy of telling a story in a soothing and validating relationship' (p.181).

## Doing this too fast or too early in the journey can be significantly unhelpful or dangerous

The problem is that to go too fast into processing traumatic memories would be like deciding to do a surgery without appropriate preparation and anaesthesia. It would cause additional pain and could be significantly destabilizing or even life threatening. There are a lot of preparations to make to ensure that any physical operation does not add to the trauma by causing further infections or crises. In the same way, the foundations need to be built over time that create a strong sense of safety and security, before the wounds of the trauma can be released from the infection and pain that is buried within them. The very nature of trauma recovery is that it is never a straight line to recovery but a journey which is wiggly and also sometimes repetitive, because the layers of trauma need to be frequently attended to as more healing comes at a greater depth.

Once emotional and physical safety and stability have been established and the child is not in a whirlwind of trauma symptoms that are interrupting their ability to cope with normal life, and the child is aware of some of the memories of past trauma that are beginning to come into their conscious memory, they need help processing these memories so they no longer negatively impact their day-to-day life.

This is the most essential element of recovery because it is the part of the journey where recovery is now noticeable. This should be led by a qualified psychologist, psychotherapist or creative psychotherapist who is trained to do so and is clinically supervised by someone who offers external insight that can be vital to the navigation towards recovery. I would suggest that a mentor, a parent, a friend, a mental health first aider or someone with any other short training would not provide the required understanding to be able to lead this process with safety and insight.

'What was going on at home was far too difficult to explain or even speak about, so people assumed I had anxiety. They just insisted I did breathing exercises and mindfulness and when I struggled to because of my past, they thought I was "non-engaging and naughty". I didn't have words to explain that when my dad went into a rage, he had pushed a pillow over my face to suffocate me and I almost died. Breathing exercises were triggering. No one knew how much my dad used to hurt me and I didn't think I could tell them.' *Jim, now aged 19, speaking about his school support*

## Fragmented trauma memories

The nature of trauma is that the experience is overwhelming and therefore too much for the person to hold as a narrative or story that is easy to tell in sequential order. The stress, overwhelm and terror of the traumatic experience causes the narrative to fragment or shatter into separate pieces, which then cause the child to feel further powerless about their own story. When memories surface, at first it can feel as if they are covered in a cloud, and the child can only just grasp them and struggle to believe that it happened to them. Then, as the memories become clearer as the cloud moves away, it becomes painful to believe it was them and their body that was hurt and this can take their breath away physically. They can want to think it didn't happen and it was a dream, because it is too awful to believe it happened to them.

Fisher (2017) describes what we see so often in the therapy room: 'individuals are left with a legacy of symptoms and reactions with no context that identifies them as memory' (p.20). As psychotherapists, we see children – often with their families present – with heightened sensitivity around safety and danger, hypervigilance around every sensory input, or they are frozen, stuck, shut down or dissociative. They may have challenges with anger or aggression, loneliness or self-hatred, anxiety, depression or suicidality, chronic shame and a terror of further abandonment. They may be asking for help because they struggle in relationships, or struggle with addictions or self-harming or disordered eating, but they may also struggle to connect past experiences with present challenging behaviours. They can seem to be in internal conflict, desperately wanting help, but when they can have this help, struggling to emotionally or physically stay in the room and engage with any of the main reasons they came to seek help. The internal turmoil can be so painful and distressing that denial of it all seems a better option, until they feel once more that they cannot cope and need to seek help again.

The fragmented pieces of memory are stored as sensory memories or body memories or feelings that are trapped, buried and stuck in time. Sometimes the trauma memories are difficult to access due to different experiences, which could be their level of shock, their age at the time of the experience or that the perpetrator used blindfolds or drugged them to stop the factual recollection of the events and so that they can avoid prosecution. This can make it difficult to remember aspects of the abuse and can feel to the survivor as if they are watching themselves on a television screen rather than it happening to them. Occasionally, a survivor may want to find films or images of such abuse to help them try and remember what happened to them because of the frustration of the dissociation and disconnection, and the need to know fully what took place. They can feel as if they are living on a constant oscillation between searching for more memories and facts of what happened and then denial and fear that it did happen.

The aim of trauma processing is that these fragments can begin to be seen, heard, validated and tended to by adults who are the empathetic witnesses of the unfolding of the trauma narrative. This can then enable the child to accept, acknowledge, own, believe and feel the pain of what happened to them without collapsing or further fragmenting.

Judith Herman describes the essential role of the therapist who has spent time building that safe attachment relationship where 'the therapist plays the role of witness and ally, in whose presence the survivor can speak the unspeakable' (2022, p.175).

Frances Waters (2016) explains that:

> having a positive relationship with the child is a prerequisite for providing the structure for trauma processing. When the therapist has capacity 'to hold' the child's intense affect, validate the child's suffering, and help the child manage it, the child builds the confidence to revisit the horrors of the past. (p.288)

For Type II and III trauma, this requires a trauma recovery focused therapist to lead and facilitate this.

## Staying within the Window of Tolerance

When the trauma processing takes place, it can cause the child to experience deep distress and their past challenges to resurface again. It is vital that the adults around the child are aware that this could happen, and everyone is able to remind themselves and the child that this is normal, it is to be expected and it does not necessarily mean that they are back to the start of the journey and that things will quickly implode.

The child should be in their Window of Tolerance at the start of the session and be able to get and keep themselves there with relative confidence in normal situations. Keeping them aware of their 'window' and how they may be shifting during the trauma processing is vital and helps them feel empowered to collaborate with their therapist. They could even point to a diagram of the Window of Tolerance as they talk, to indicate how they are feeling if the words are too difficult to access. It's important to keep them within that Window of Tolerance because the processing cannot happen if they are flooded or overwhelmed with emotions or memories.

If the child is too shocked or not able to return to a state of relative calm soon after the sessions, then the therapist needs to slow down again and go back to safety and stabilization work until there is enough strength for the child to continue. When there is increased safety and stability, the child can then be enabled to review small elements of the trauma story that have already been shared, using tools to help them stay in their Window of Tolerance and feel supported and safe. The plan is that as the therapeutic work progresses, the Window of Tolerance becomes larger and larger because they feel safer for longer.

## Assessing the timing

It is vital that the therapist who leads this stage of the recovery journey is able to assess if the child is ready. The child should have the following in place:

- An attachment relationship with someone who is prepared and understands what the process could look like in terms of shock, pain and relief.
- A toolbox of therapeutic tools to use that have become familiar and help bring comfort, calm and relief in the face of overwhelming emotional dysregulation.
- A safety plan co-created to remind the child what they can do if they move into a sudden flow of new memories that could threaten to interrupt their sleep or play.
- A therapist to lead on this process (psychotherapist, psychologist,

counsellor, creative therapist), who is trained in trauma recovery in all areas covered in this book and has experience doing this successfully with other children.

It is important to note that when a child has previously not expressed emotions and now has greater understanding of them, they may demonstrate increased expression as they process the trauma. They usually don't stay like this, but it is a transition period of adjustment to a greater range of emotional expression and a greater need to express emotion. If the adults around them make space, validate and soothe the child, they will eventually need to be less demonstrative and expressive, and life may feel calmer.

## Support in the home
It is also vital that the child senses that the parent or carer will be able to know the story without it impacting them in a way that causes family stress. The way that the primary attachment figure responds to the story of the traumatic experience is important, and the way they express support in their tone of voice, facial expression and body language is central to the child's healing and ongoing relationship. Silberg (2012) explains how it is helpful to 'prepare the parent or caregiver to listen nondefensively' because 'children need to know that their parents are strong enough to handle the intense affect and grief that accompanies the trauma' (p.194).

## The SAFE model
Here is a simple model that I created to help all ages process trauma in a safer way. Once they have some safety and stability and a trauma memory is now being interruptive to their life, surfacing as a flashback, nightmare or memory, it needs to be processed.

My simple processing model is sequential and helps make sure that the time spent processing is not dysregulating or distressing. It uses the word SAFE to help both professionals and the traumatized person themselves remember the order of how to work through a painful memory.

## THE SAFE MODEL

**S** Seen - who knows you and cares?
Safe - where do you feel safe?
Spot your reactions to things.

**A** Acknowledge what happened.
Acknowledge some of your feelings.

**F** Focus on something hopeful.
Find a passion to throw yourself into.

**E** Expect a wiggly journey.
Encourage yourself.
Externalize not internalize.

THE SAFE MODEL © BETSY DE THIERRY 2025

**TRFM® TOOL 10: The SAFE model**

## It starts with S

Here is the starting point and time to reflect, write, draw or speak about these kinds of areas:

- Who are you SEEN and known by?
- Which part of you is feeling distress right now – the V, I or P?
- How would you describe the ways that you feel emotionally SAFE right now?
- SPOT the reactions you may have been having when this memory was bubbling up?
- Remember that there is NO SHAME in what you are feeling because this trauma never should have happened to you and it wasn't your fault.

Seen by someone
Seen as VIP
Safe emotionally
Spot the reactions/feelings
Shame reduces

### Then we go to A

- Can you ACKNOWLEDGE some of what has happened?
- Can you ACKNOWLEDGE some of the feelings you have felt?
- Take your time here and stay within your Window of Tolerance. If you feel yourself move out of that space of being 'okay', then quickly move to F.

Acknowledge some of what's happened.
Acknowledge some of the feelings.

### Then we go to F

This process is important to be able to ground yourself in how well you are doing and who is on the journey supporting you. There is a point to going through this pain — it is so that life will be less painful, and you can be less interrupted as you develop your passions.

Focus on some positives and some hope.
Find a passion and purpose.

### Finally, we land at E

Here you remind yourself that it is not meant to be a quick and easy journey, and many people aren't strong enough to do this — so well done! You can encourage yourself and remember the positive elements of recovery so far. Try and externalize the latest step in your journey, whether through art or writing or through chatting to a friend or supporter.

Expect it to be a wiggly journey!
Encourage yourself at every tiny move!
Externalize as much as possible in a safe way.

This SAFE model work can be done with a supportive adult, carefully, at the pace that the child sets. Eventually, older children can do it on their own when they feel triggered, distressed or anxious about something. It is a model that is easy to remember and enables safe processing that is not overwhelming due to the sequence of the stages.

## Trauma processing

A central stage of the recovery process is about processing the trauma. This can, of course, only happen once the child has been helped to find some kind of stability and has been able to experience consistent relationships in which they have begun to recognize the feelings of being safe. They also need to have learned some self-regulation and comfort strategies, having experienced consistent co-regulation with a key attachment figure or two, begun to learn to feel some everyday feelings and sensations, and started to be curious about themselves. Then they are safe enough to begin to allow memories to surface. If memories surface before these important stages have been secured, then it is harder to stop the memories creating complete chaos, but it is not completely impossible to work on all the areas simultaneously. It is important to note what Putnam (1997) worded so well: 'Transforming traumatic experiences may also involve facilitating autonomy, control, and competence in ways that do not need to directly acknowledge the role of trauma in constricting or distortion these functions' (p.286).

The trauma needs processing with the help of a psychotherapist who knows how to carefully lead the child through, making sure that things don't move too fast and safety is always monitored. The emotions accompanying the memories can be massive and feel overwhelming to the child and everyone around them, and so it is important to work carefully with the right foundations of relationship, safety and stability.

## Integrative narrative

An integrative narrative is the ability to be able to tell the story of the trauma, without it being overwhelming or emotionless. A child cannot speak about what has happened while they are in shock or numb or in some way disconnected to their own experiences. Therefore, one of the signs of their progression towards recovery is the ability for the child to speak of their story with some order, appropriate emotion, expressions of the sense of injustice, realization that it was wrong that it happened and a feeling of deep sadness or shock or anger or any other emotion that they can acknowledge. In the presence of the therapist who validates and witnesses this story unfolding, the child can then begin to order the story and emotions alongside the ways that they coped. The trauma symptoms, defence mechanisms and coping methods can be named and validated as helping them stay alive in the face of terror, powerlessness and overwhelm.

Sometimes, after a long time receiving therapy, the child may find it helpful to draw a timeline of their life and put the positive experiences, friendships and events on the top of the timeline and the negative ones at the bottom. This gives a sense of their story visually, with colours and pictures to help them express what they have been through and what helped them.

This integrative narrative brings together the work of the child and the therapist and is the culmination of the deep explorations of what happened and how they coped and how they now feel. This needs to not be rushed but takes time, probably more than a year of regular therapy for Type II trauma or two years for Type III trauma, if the child's home is now a place of safety and they have longer-term attachment relationships. Herman (2022) explains that 'Richard Mollica describes the transformed trauma story as simply "a new story" which is "no longer about shame and humiliation" but rather "about dignity and virtue". Through their storytelling, his refugee patients "regain the world they have lost"' (p.181).

The integrative narrative is a sign that the main sting and turmoil of the story have now been healed, leaving the child with knowledge of what has happened and an awareness of how they coped and how they can now move forward with more healthy coping mechanisms.

I often say that integrity comes from integration. For a person to be able to have integrity, they need to become integrated in their conscious and subconscious as the trauma is processed and there are no secrets left in the darkness of their soul. Trauma causes a person to keep secrets from themselves due to the nature of the terror, power-lessness and overwhelm. When trauma recovery is complete, they are less likely to demonstrate conflicting values and behaviours and are able to feel a sense of wholeness. They may sometimes still feel as if the story of their life is like a dream, but they know it is true.

When any of us are in a position of witnessing some element of a person's story or the coming together of several parts of a story, we need to recognize and honour the privilege. Brené Brown (2024) has written: 'We have been entrusted with something valuable that we should treat with respect and care. We are good stewards of the stories we hear by listening, being curious, affirming and believing people when they tell us how they experienced something.'

## Grief

It is vital to note that grief can become present and powerful as the trauma is processed. The question 'Why did it have to be me?' has to be asked and validated. The feelings of grief and loss need to be validated as the child feels the pain of the injustice. The child needs to know that the parents or carer can contain the grief and loss, and not fall into deep shame and guilt which stops the important stage of mourning over what was lost. Healthy mourning over past trauma does come to a place of rest, where it is not as powerful or emotional and is instead a gentle sense of peace as the child becomes able to close that chapter and open a new one. The cry from the depth of a child's heart can be 'Why did no one rescue me or stop this?' We need to be able to hold that space and contain their pain so that they feel validated and cared for, and we need to share the same sense of deep injustice about what has happened to them.

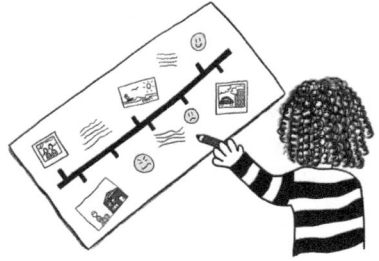

## Identity building and self-concept

As the child processes the trauma, they will begin to realize that some of their interests and hobbies could be due to trying to survive. They may need to reflect on who they are now as they begin to see their lives from the perspective of trauma survival. Their passion for self-defence or interest in helping younger children or commitment to fitness could all point to that primitive need to stay alive and stop it happening to other children. Mearns and Cooper (2005) explain how trauma can disrupt 'the whole assumptive frame upon which our sense of self is founded' (p.65).

The child may realize that they are not 'naughty' and they don't have 'trouble concentrating' and they are not 'defiant or angry', but that these behaviours are symptoms of the distress that was hidden from many. As they process the behaviour and emotional expression that their identity may be formed by, they are able to recognize that this is not *who* they are but *how they survived*. This gives them the opportunity to explore what they really enjoy now that they are not needing to be defensive and hypervigilant to further stress and terror. This process needs to be an intentional element of the trauma processing, which is supported by the parents or carer, who may find it a surprise that the child discovers a new interest, passion or sense of identity. As the child grows through the trauma recovery process, they can view themselves as a strong survivor who did well with what tools they had, but this is the time for them now to be empowered to become who they want to become. Some children will need support as they explore what interests they have and what skills they would like to develop as they begin a new fresh chapter of their lives with a firmer foundation.

Self-loathing, self-hatred and low self-esteem can be trauma symptoms that are intertwined with the shame of the experiences that wounded them and impacted their sense of self. As the child processes the trauma, they can be taught to see themselves as survivors who are courageous and powerful. They can be helped to write self-affirmations that feel authentic in the moment of realizing how far they have come in learning that what happened to them was not their fault and that they were incredible at using coping mechanisms that helped them survive what may have felt unsurvivable.

Society seems to be committed to persuading children to make long-term decisions about who they are, while those of us who have spent decades working with children recognize that it is normal for them to 'go through phases' and change their mind. I don't see many adults committed to being superheroes with a cape, and yet many children under 8 assume that is what their future holds. As the supportive adults, we need to be relaxed and let the child explore and try new things, while recognizing that they may change their mind and choose some different passions. That is childhood, and we need to be committed to that level of flexibility.

## Different tools that help process memories

There are some different tools that help process the trauma, and these can be helpful when the other elements of trauma recovery have been explored. To rush to have six or ten weeks of therapy for fast trauma processing when the foundations for the child's relationships and environments have not been built can be counterproductive in the long term. If they are rushed to 'recover', then the child may feel further disempowered and create a part of them that pleases the adult and seems recovered, while another part or parts of them hold the trauma memories and symptoms away from view. This would only become apparent when they are older.

Therapy is the method for trauma processing to be able to keep the child safe in the face of the overwhelming experiences, memories, symptoms of distress and internal chaos that can feel volcanic or frozen in time.

There is a wide range of therapy trainings, many of which specialize in one of the areas of impact that are explored in Section 2: the body, the emotions, the subconscious, the mind, and relationships. The therapist needs to have skill and training in each of these areas so that they can confidently lead the child through the difficult areas where memories, both sensory, body, mind or fragments of each, can be slowly invited to be seen, heard, validated and finally processed to discharge the turmoil, shock and pain. This has to take place in small doses so that the child doesn't become further overwhelmed and is able to stay safe and have supportive relationships that enable the stability and safety to continue all week around the therapy sessions.

'When I started therapy, I was in trouble all the time because I couldn't sit still and used to get into fights. I didn't want to, and I wanted to be good but somehow I would just get irritated and would lash out. I ended up with no friends really and I was sad, but that made me angrier. So, I was always in trouble. When I understood that I wasn't a bad kid but was actually angry that my dad had left, it all made sense. I now know why I do stuff and can do other things instead when my feelings get too big for me. I am calmer now and sleep better too. I am beginning to make good friends again.' *Paul, aged 12*

## Conclusion

Processing the trauma is the tough element of recovery. Many children will happily play therapeutic games, learn neuroscience, do art activities and enjoy the nurturing company of an adult while fiercely avoiding any mention of the trauma experience that they had to endure. They can be clever to distract the adult and keep a strong boundary around the memories, which can create a shared anxiety about the story of trauma. When the adult recognizes that avoidance is a natural response, they must remain aware that for the child to recover from the horrors of what took place, they need to be supported to be courageous enough to gently bring it into the time they share. The pace needs to be carefully considered, with continual evaluation of the child's safety, stability and trauma symptoms.

## Questions to reflect on
### For parents/carers/therapeutic mentors

- Can you reflect on how far the child has come in their journey and if they are safe enough now to process the trauma memories?
- Can you recognize that the child is able to now use tools to help them feel safe and get back into the Window of Tolerance?
- Can the child use words to describe some of what happened without shame making them laugh, avoid the real elements, minimalize or be sarcastic?
- Has the child got a trauma therapist to help them process some of the memories in a way that is safe?
- Have you tried to use the SAFE model in your own trauma processing?
- How has the child changed over the time of recovery? Has this impacted their identity? How are you finding that challenge of not holding too tightly to any of their passions, hobbies, opinions or views as they change because the trauma has less impact on them?
- Have you heard them tell their integrative narrative or have you seen a timeline or any artwork that seems to summarize where they were and where they are not? Have you managed to validate and affirm the courage that they have shown on this journey?

### For therapists

- What training and tools do you have for processing trauma? Have you worked within a whole trauma recovery model before, like my model, where time is spent building safety and positive home attachments, and upskilling the parents and carers, alongside the trauma processing? What would you change about how you work?

- How would your work change now you have explored these elements that include recovery from the trauma impact on the body, emotions, mind, relationships and unconscious? What do you feel competent in and what do you need to train in further?

# SECTION 3

# DIFFERENT TRAUMATIC EXPERIENCES

This section looks at the different traumatic experiences that could have happened to each child and therefore what specific symptoms could have developed to enable the child to survive those experiences. The recovery journey will need to start at the safety and stabilization stage, which is explored in Section 1, and then they will need to begin to explore the impact of the trauma on their body, mind, emotions, relationships and eventually their subconscious, as detailed in Section 2. During this stage of the recovery process, the specific trauma experience needs to be explored. Each child will have had a different experience of trauma with a different setting, and will be a different personality who views their different combination of traumatic experiences. No one child's experience is the same, but there is a sense of similarity of the elements of the journey and also of the specific symptoms that are common to each type of traumatic experience. This is a section that is not meant to be read as a whole if you are a parent or carer, so that you can focus on the child you are caring for. You can look up the chapter titles and explore what you think may have happened to them. If you are a professional, then obviously this is important for the work you do with the range of children and young people that you support. The first chapter in this section will explore grief, a central aspect in the impact of trauma, and so would be relevant to most of the children who have experienced trauma.

## The areas that will be explored

The overall areas in this section are grief, sexual trauma, physical abuse, medical trauma, emotional abuse and organizational trauma.

Emotional neglect and collective trauma are the focus of two of my separate books and there is not enough space here to rewrite those. *The Simple Guide to Emotional Neglect* (2023) explores the impact and recovery from the experience of a child who had busy working parents who couldn't spend much time in emotional connection, through to the experience of a child who spent hours alone or in a large group and felt abandoned, rejected, uncared for and unloved. *The Simple Guide to Collective Trauma* (2021) explores the impact and recovery from different experiences such as COVID, knife attack, war, earthquake or natural disaster of any kind. It is different from an experience that one person endures and so the recovery journey is also different.

# CHAPTER 17

# Grief, Loss and Change

When loss is the central issue, the child may express fear or behaviours that are based on the terror of losing someone else or something else. Grief may impact the child's body, emotions, mind, relationships or subconscious, and the previous chapters explore that, but there are other elements of their experience that need to be noted and supported.

Whenever there is trauma, there is always grief because loss is always experienced when the wound of trauma is present, and the child has always lost something. In Brené Brown's (2021) exploration of grief, she quotes Neimeyer: 'a central process in grieving is the attempt to reaffirm or reconstruct a world of meaning that has been challenged by loss' (p.110). She then continues with an exploration of her research where three main elements of grief emerged from the data, which were loss, longing and feeling lost. 'The losses being the loss of normality, the loss of what could be, and the loss of what we thought we knew or understood about something or someone' (p.110). While the research was with adults, the themes are similar with children who are grieving due to loss.

## Bereavement

A child who has experienced the death of a loved one, especially a parent or sibling, can feel anxious about the other relationships that they value. Unlike other trauma experiences, with grief it can be helpful to talk about the person that they miss. With the experience of bereavement, the child and family often feel able to calmly and easily explain that they may be feeling deeply sad, whereas in other experiences of trauma, there can be the powerful feeling of shame that stops the ability to use words easily. In bereavement, the child usually has the empathy of those around them due to being able to easily express what has happened, unlike other traumatic experiences that remain unspoken. But bereavement can cause fear-related behaviours where the child needs reassurance about the location and health of their loved ones. They may feel less able to take risks or commit themselves to future plans because they feel overwhelmed by trying to survive the risks of their present day to day. They may spend more time in books, online games or other ways to avoid the reality of their present situation because the loss of their loved one is too hard to hold in the conscious, and denial or dissociation feels safer. They may feel as if they have a duty to make their loved one proud of them, and so they may 'throw themselves' into work or a hobby with a new level of commitment or passion.

Bereavement can impact sleep and cause restlessness, and sometimes cause a fear of going to sleep, in case they 'slip into death', especially if they have seen a person that they love looking as if they are sleeping when they were in fact deceased. Bereavement can impact a child's ability to learn in school as they struggle to focus on what can feel to them like irrelevant subjects when they feel so deeply sad and their life seems to have paused. They may be more sensitive, more reactive or more dissociative. Other children can be kind but can also get bored and show less kindness and compassion when a child is sad a few weeks after the loss of a loved one. This can lead to their friendships sometimes being less supportive and the child feeling lonelier, which can exacerbate the feelings of loss.

Children grieve slightly differently from adults. They can feel deeply sad one moment and then be distracted by something and forget the sadness. It can be confusing for the adults around them unless it is understood. Winston's Wish, a bereavement charity in the UK, describes the difference beautifully:

> Adults can often feel overwhelmed by grief, as if they are caught in the current of a river and find it hard to get out. Whereas young children in particular, tend to 'jump' in and out of their grief – a little like jumping in and out of a puddle – leaping from feeling very upset and distressed

one moment to wanting to know what's for tea or whether they can play football, for example. The reason for this is that children need a break from the powerful emotions that accompany their grief and so are able to jump out of them for a while in order that they are not overwhelmed. (Winston's Wish, 2020)

## Loss of pets

It is worth noting that children can have a deep sense of grief about losing a pet. The death of a pet can be felt deeply, especially if they had their animal as an attachment relationship where they shared secrets and worries. The child needs to have this loss validated, and when the pet was a friendship and attachment, they will need support as they navigate the feelings of sadness and shock.

## Ambiguous loss

This is the confusing experience of loss where the person may feel stuck in grief which is sometimes not validated because the person that they are grieving has not permanently 'gone'; they haven't died but they are in some ways inaccessible or less accessible. This can leave the child or adult in a state of turmoil because they usually are less able to speak about it, and if they do, there can be less empathy and less support, and the process of grief seems to freeze in time.

The kind of experiences of ambiguous loss can include:

- parents divorcing
- moving area or country
- a parent going to prison
- a parent in the military stationed away from home
- a sibling leaving the home longer term
- a loved one becoming a missing person.

Children of all ages can struggle to express their feelings about ambiguous grief because they either feel shame or doubt that there would be sufficient empathy and kindness to warrant the emotional energy to attempt to express how they feel.

## Divorce or parental separation

When a child has to process the change of family experience, they can sometimes grieve the past and grieve what they wanted to have. Sometimes children are able to quickly 'bounce back' and may even be able to reframe the change as a positive one with more presents, more homes and more treats. There are some good therapeutic story books that tell the story of children or animals who have experienced their parents divorcing, and these are helpful to use to explore how the characters of the story are feeling and what they are thinking. When we use stories of others, it can help the children feel that their own feelings and reactions of sadness or confusion or anger are validated and therefore don't need to be hidden.

Others hide their feelings of disappointment, which can be seen as behaviours that may be either hyperaroused or hypoaroused, and these indicate the child's need to spend time with those they love to feel safe, seen, heard, validated and cared for. They may need time to talk and process their thoughts. Younger children tend to process in short bursts and play out some of what they are feeling through their normal play with toys. Older children and teenagers can prefer to spend time engaging in a favourite activity with their parent, with time to talk about it and have space for any questions or reflections.

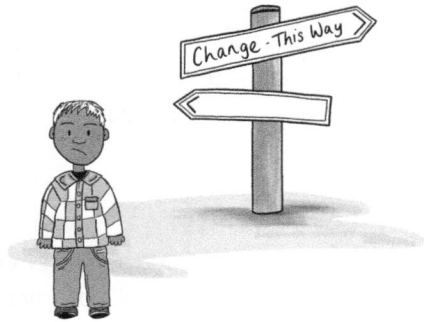

## New school/home/area/country

Change requires emotional energy and can be something that many people avoid. The change of a new school or area can be full of hope and feel exciting, alongside provoking feelings of fear. The preparation for change is important to help the transition. It is also helpful to validate the reality that many humans can struggle with change. When a child is empowered to make some decisions about the colour of paint in their bedroom or if they can have a new duvet cover, then they feel less powerless and more part of the collaboration of the move. It's important to get the balance of involving them enough that they don't feel left out and not involving them to the extent that they feel responsible for things going well or feel overwhelmed by the details. Getting that detail right helps the transition seem less traumatic and more exciting, despite the loss that they may feel. If it is a major change for the child, such as a new culture, then it is best to try and help them have some small experiences of those new cultural aspects if possible, whether that is the new type of clothing, food, accents, behaviour or rules.

Sometimes they may suddenly feel the loss of the country, home or school after they have settled in a little bit and the novelty has worn off. When they express that loss, they need to be helped to feel it rather than be distracted from it, so that they can have these feelings validated before they can be reminded of anything positive that they now have in their life.

'I know it may sound strange, but I just miss my home. Nothing is the same as that place. I guess that's where I felt at home and now I feel like I'm always just visiting.' *Andrew, aged 14*

## Move to kinship care/foster care/residential care

I write this very much aware of how much The System is currently failing these children on so many levels. There are so many excellent professionals trying their best with limited time and budget to be able to work in the way they want to. I hear of horrific stories of vulnerable children having to make sudden transitions, with distressing details where the child's needs are not validated in any way. There are also many, many incredible professionals within the field fighting hard to bring in change and demonstrating authentic care for families. We need to continue to fight for The System to become more trauma informed urgently and we must keep supporting each other working with the most vulnerable in our society.

Moving the child from one 'home' to another, with different adults taking on responsibility for their care is the kind of change and transition that requires significant planning to reduce any potential trauma. The child needs to be empowered to make some suggestions about what they would like to take with them, what is important for them to have and whatever else they would like to be able to feel heard.

The child will need to adjust, find out what it is like and may simulta-neously feel big feelings such as confusion, rejection, abandonment, shame, turmoil and deep disappointment. These feelings may not be able to be expressed for some time due to the change and their need to assess how safe they are, and so may be noticed as symptoms of distress in behaviour or other emotions that are easier to feel and express such as anger, boredom, irritation or the need to withdraw.

The greatest need the child will probably have will be for relation-ships that offer stability, safety and reassurance and any other aspects of life that can be predictable and feel familiar. This loss and grief can be an additional challenge to a child who has already experienced trauma and therefore may have defence mechanisms and coping methods which will be utilized to help them keep going. They may seem to be 'coping well' and even say that they are 'just fine'. What we recognize is that despite how they manage to survive the challenge, often hid-den from the view of those around them, they can feel an increase of overwhelm and desperation for stability and ease. Vulnerability is often something that they work hard to hide due to the terror of being further hurt, rejected or violated. They need all the relational care that is explored in the rest of this book.

## Homelessness

It is clear that to be homeless can be a significant trauma for anyone of any age. It is a devastating and destabilizing experience which can cause the person to feel disconnected, unvalued, bereft and alone, and all of these feelings can be shrouded with deep feelings of shame. The shame is connected to the feeling that they now don't belong 'anywhere', which can be a terrifying experience of vulnerability and powerlessness. This can cause them to feel a sense of resignation, sur-render and submission, where they have no energy to even feel the injustice of their life anymore, or they can be agitated and angry with others because of what they have suffered that has caused them to feel so rejected and abandoned. The shame can cause the person who has become homeless to wonder why it has happened to them and what they did so wrong to be left so unable to feel safe. Not 'belonging' to a home where they have a place to keep some special memories and familiar comforting objects can feel like a profound crisis and injustice.

The child may need to have photos and objects that they decide are special in school with their name on, so that they feel a stronger sense of belonging to a community which can 'hold' something that they trust them to care for.

## Other losses

Other losses and separations from loved ones are wide ranging and can include a parent being in prison, a parent working away from home for a long time, perhaps in the military, a parent who was once emotionally engaged and present and is now unwell or less able to play. These changes and losses can be difficult to grieve due to the loyalty to the parent and desire not to add further stress to their situation. This means that they can be hidden, and the child's behaviour can instead reflect their compliance or desire to help and not cause further difficulty, or they may express any behaviour which is a normal symptom of distress, as explored in the previous sections.

## The impact of loss

- Feeling disconnected or alone.
- Feeling disorientated or confused.
- Feeling destabilized and wobbly.
- Feeling exhausted, as there are constant 'first times' in the new season.
- Wondering about what life could have been like had the loss not occurred.
- Feeling sad, devastated, upset, angry or a sense of injustice about the change to their life.
- Feeling tired because of the emotions and change that they need to keep processing.
- Thinking back to 'before' the loss as more perfect than it was in reality.
- Daydreaming about the loss.
- Feeling angry with other children who have what they have lost, especially if they don't seem to appreciate it.
- Finding that learning can either be a good distraction or is

difficult to concentrate or focus on when their inner world seems so unsettled.

- Feeling anxious about what could go wrong or what changes could be coming up.
- Wanting to control their life to avoid further pain and turmoil.
- Showing different symptoms of trauma in hyperaroused or hypoaroused behaviour.

## Ideas to help the child who is grieving the loss of a loved one

The child needs to have time and ways to remember the loved one or favourite pet, with the support of a caring adult, where the child can look at photos of them, make pictures of them doing their favourite things, tell stories about them and feel fully able to dwell on how wonderful they were and how deeply sad they feel. Some children like to create a memory box full of special memories of the loved one, which they can look back through when they need to feel close to them. Some children can create a photo book that they can spend time looking through when they miss them.

It is important that they have time to ask questions about where they are and what happened, and the answers need to be as truthful as possible while being aware of the child's age and what the consequences of knowing could be. The language used is important; terms such as 'passing away' or 'sleeping' to describe death can cause confusion in young children who may form a dislike or fear of bedtime and sleeping.

It is important to make space for the child to cry and be sad without any unhelpful comments that seek to stop the crying. We need to use words to validate and affirm the reality of their feelings with facial reactions and a tone of voice that shows empathy – words such as 'Yes, it so sad, isn't it?' and 'I am gutted for you'. We need to avoid trying to help them 'move on' and therefore we should not use sentences such as 'You need to get on with your life and move on'. The child needs to be able to feel the feelings rather than push them down as this can cause future explosions or implosions. If they get stuck in a state of overwhelm with crying and feeling increasingly hopeless, then it is important to distract them in the short term and move them into doing something more comforting or positive. The adult needs to monitor this so that they are not hurried or stopped from expressing feelings of grief, but they also aren't left to dwell for too long and become helpless and hopeless. They need us to hold the safe boundaries.

Helpful therapeutic story books to read:

- *The Heart and the Bottle* by Oliver Jeffers (2010). HarperCollins Children's Books.
- *The Hare-Shaped Hope* by John Dougherty (2023). Frances Lincoln Children's Books.
- *Ollie the Octopus Loss and Bereavement Activity Book* by Karen Treisman (2021). Jessica Kingsley Publishers.
- *Badger's Parting Gifts* by Susan Varley (2013). Anderson Press.

## Conclusion

Grief and loss can cause long-term feelings of sadness, numbness, loss of enthusiasm for things that were once enjoyed, and other symptoms, but with time it does lesson. Positive relationships can enable the child to reflect, process and begin to understand more of how life looks with the changes, and so they are more able to move forward. It is possible to recover from grief, but recovery does not mean that the child will not want and need to talk about the person, the country, the school or whatever else they are missing, and we need to make space for them to explore those feelings. We need to be able to recognize that when a child is stuck in grief, they will continue to show behaviours that are outside the Window of Tolerance, rather than see these decreasing. These indicators help us know that they are beginning to recover from the shock and turmoil of the loss and move towards being able to acknowledge and accept the changes. As we support children through grief, they can feel able to learn, play and grow with less confusion and conflict.

# CHAPTER 18

# Sexual Trauma

Sexual trauma is devastating. This chapter could be hard to read for any adult who has experienced any kind of sexual abuse in their past. All trauma that is inflicted on the physical body impacts more than just the body, and sexual trauma is a violation that seems to transcend the realm of just physical harm and relational harm and is a deep wound that causes shame and turmoil to the survivor. The sexual area of the body is sometimes referred to as a person's 'private parts', and that description helps bring to light the reason that sexual trauma causes such a terrifying violation. Sexual abuse is a physical, emotional and relational trauma that exposes and harms the private, most intimate and unseen area of a person's body that children and adults seek to keep covered. The recovery route needs to start at the stages explored in Sections 1 and 2 of this book so that the general foundation of safety and stability is laid to build recovery on, alongside the general areas of the child's life that are impacted by all trauma. This chapter then focuses on the themes that develop to survive sexual abuse, which need to be explored for recovery to be found.

## Sexual abuse

Sexual abuse can happen to anyone, and it is not just the touching of a child's genital area but also other aspects of violation that impact a child. It is terrifying, overwhelming and shocking for a child and can have long-term impact unless they are helped to recover.

> Child sexual abuse is any interaction between a child and an adult (or another child) in which the child is used for the sexual stimulation of the perpetrator or an observer. Sexual abuse can include both touching

and non-touching behaviours. Non-touching behaviours can include voyeurism (trying to look at a child's naked body), exhibitionism, or exposing the child to pornography. Children of all ages, races, ethnicities, and economic backgrounds may experience sexual abuse. Child sexual abuse affects both girls and boys in all kinds of neighbourhoods and communities. (National Child Traumatic Stress Network, n.d.)

Sexual abuse can be a one-off experience that impacts the child long term if they are unable to tell anyone, and this is sometimes called molestation. It can also be something that occurs more frequently, and the child can know and be familiar with the perpetrator and so no one seems suspicious about what is happening. The child can feel trapped in the secret that they have been told to keep and what may happen if they tell anyone. It can be hard for a child to tell someone else due to feeling shame that it is probably their own fault and they are 'naughty' or 'dirty'. Or the child may feel scared of how others may react if they knew what happened and they may worry about what could happen next. Often the child 'buries' the memories immediately for fear of 'getting told off' or being blamed for what happened. Every story of sexual abuse is unique, and each one is damaging, but restoring the child to a place where they don't feel terror, sadness, shame, turmoil, confusion or dirty about what has happened is entirely possible and essential.

## Male sexual abuse
While a lot of the historic research around sexual abuse has been predominately around females as victims, it needs to be noted that males can also be victims. 'Male sexual abuse is any unwanted or non-consensual sexual act performed against a male adult or child at any time in his life' (NHS England, 2022). There are many reasons why sexual abuse is not reported to the police, and for males this can include fears around how they may be viewed and if they would be believed, alongside 'fears that their sexuality could become the focus of any investigation' (Badenoch, 2015). Boys may be afraid that what they experienced was not abuse as their physiological reactions seemed to indicate a conflict of emotion, with them seeming to be curious and excited about the sexual experience yet also feeling unable to run away, hide or refuse to comply.

A lack of knowledge regarding the physiologic reaction to attack and the fact that erection or orgasm can occur even in traumatic situations may contribute to this belief. This false notion may not only prevent people from believing that men may be abused, but it may also prevent men from recognizing victimization when it does. (Thomas & Kopel, 2023)

For many survivors of male sexual abuse, the shame and secrecy of what has happened can feel intensely life altering as they try and pretend that nothing has happened while simultaneously experiencing conflicting feelings and emotions about themselves, their masculinity, vulnerability and sexuality.

## Rape

Rape can be an element of sexual abuse and it can also be experienced as a one-off traumatic event that can shatter the person's sense of safety and innocence. The USA's Federal Bureau of Investigation defines rape in a widely used definition as the 'penetration, no matter how slight, of the vagina or anus with any body part or object, or penetration by a sex organ of another person, without the victim's consent' (Federal Bureau of Investigation, 2017). In 1972, a psychiatric nurse and a sociologist embarked on a study of the psychological effects of rape by spending a year working in the emergency room of Boston City Hospital and interviewing any child or adult who was a victim of rape. They noted the trauma symptoms which followed, and they are those that we still see today in our therapy rooms after rape and sexual assault. They were 'insomnia, nausea, startle responses, and nightmares, as well as dissociative or numbing symptoms' (Burgess & Holmstrom, 1974).

The impact of rape is devastating on many levels. Herman (2022) asserts that the 'The rapist's purpose is to terrorize, dominate, and humiliate the victim' (p.58). The person is left shocked, feeling shattered and changed. The world seems altered and different from that moment onwards. The experience is one of terror, powerlessness and total overwhelm, to the extent that the victim can often question after the event if they are still alive in any way. The memory is often almost completely fragmented into pieces, of the pain, the sounds, smells, feelings and the utter devastation, turmoil and confusion. It is an experience that can cause immediate shock, horror and terror, and be difficult to begin to describe in words because 'the victim does not experience rape as sexual in nature, but rather as a confrontation with death' (Mezey & Taylor, 1988; Burgess & Holmstrom, 1974).

## The automatic survival reaction

One of the factors that can cause shame and/or guilt to develop is the question that many are left with regarding their automatic reaction to freeze. Often the rape survivor cannot understand why they didn't run, shout, scream, hit, kick or run to the nearest person afterwards, crying and screaming. Following the rape, many people don't manage to run to safety and ask for support, but instead 'keep going' with daily life while they struggle with symptoms of shock and horror. Adults in positions of trust need to understand that when a child doesn't immediately tell anyone or ask for help and when they were unable to run away, fight or scream, that is a normal human response to an utterly horrific and terrifying experience and demonstrates how bad it was. Every child needs reassurance that their response is a normal one to something that was so deeply frightening. Children can recognize their lack of physical strength in comparison to an adult, which increases their sense of powerlessness and overwhelm as they instinctively realize that they are unable to fight or flight. This results in the common automatic survival response of freezing and dissociating in order to stay alive. Often the scream they thought came through their mouth was actually an internal scream, and the freeze reaction resulted in further physical pain.

## Organized sexual abuse led by adults

Although many people might want to pretend that organized sexual abuse doesn't take place, sadly that is not the case, and it needs to be noted that there are networks of adults who strategize to abuse children for their own pleasure and to generate finance.

Sexual exploitation is a type of sexual abuse where the adult manipulates or deceives the child into sexual activity, either online or in person, and they are given gifts, drugs, money or something that they need such as attention or belonging in exchange. The challenge of this is that the adult or older perpetrator may appear to be a kind and attentive friend and the sexual activity may look fully consensual when it is not. When a child is manipulated into this abuse, it is called grooming.

Some children are trafficked across the country or into a different country for sexual exploitation, and sometimes violence can be used.

Some children are made to abuse other children or adults and are left feeling that they are bad people who do awful things, without being able to see that they were manipulated, controlled and terrified of refusing to do what they were told.

Sometimes groups or gangs of people of different ages have sexual abuse as an element of their normal activities, which can lead to new victims complying while wondering why others are not complaining.

Sometimes this abuse can involve groups of perpetrators and can involve physical harm or torture, and due to the nature of this abuse, the child can be blindfolded or drugged in order to ensure that evidence won't be easily accessible. This experience can lead to confusion and stress when adults who support children want to ask questions about what they endured, because the child may not have easy answers and the memories will probably be fragmented into emotions, body memories and shock, with few visual memories.

## Non-consensual peer sex and sexual exploitation

A challenge for many young people is that they may not be fully sure if what they experienced was sexual abuse or rape because there can be confusion regarding the concept of consent. Research has found that young people have not been able to understand what consent is because they had understood that any refusal around sexual activity would be communicated with a clear verbal 'no', 'unlike other forms of human interaction where declining is typically much less direct' (Coy et al., 2013, p.9). This research found that both consent and coercion 'are slippery concepts, making the drawing of such boundaries complex and even contradictory' (p.11). They argue that 13–14-year-olds are less likely to recognize non-consensual sex compared to other age groups. Therefore, a conclusion that can be drawn is that many young people have experienced sexual activity that was not fully consented to or where they felt confused, scared or coerced. The impact of that could be profound, causing emotional and physical turmoil that may seem to them to have no reason and could make them feel that they are 'not okay' or 'something is wrong' or 'they are struggling with their mental health', but where they cannot see the correlation of their experience and the resulting impact.

Research has evidenced that gangs are contexts 'where masculinity is often enacted through violence' (Coy *et al.*, 2013, p.69). In this context, young women can be interpreted as 'sexually available' if they dress or act in certain ways.

> The connection we found between the two is the concept of 'man points', which can be accrued through sexual conquest. Sexually exploitative activity can be subsequently framed as the fault of young women. Young men's decisions thus appear invisible outside of the gang, while inside they are of central importance in establishing status and authority. For young women, pressure to avoid being labelled 'frigid' and the limited roles in which they are cast gives little space for resisting expectations of sexual availability. (Coy *et al.*, 2013, p.69)

Girls express how powerless they can feel to blame or name calling. If they meet up with a man, wear specific clothes or are unable to use words to express their opinions or boundaries, that can be used as evidence for any sexual experience that they said they didn't want, and if they don't comply, they can be harassed and called names. Often young people who have been sexually exploited tell us that they thought it was their fault and they had made bad choices, and they are unaware that they have been victims. Young people today are navigating a maze of expectation around sexual norms that is fuelled by the internet and a lack of adults available to answer questions and facilitate reflection, often due to lack of funding around mentors and sexual education since it is not seen as a global priority to help their mental health and wellbeing.

## Pornography and social media

Pornography is a crucial element of the sexual abuse field, and a widely cited definition is 'sexually explicit media that are primarily intended to sexually arouse the audience' (Malamuth, 2001). With the increase of access to the internet and the use of social media, it is not hard for children to find easy pornographic images. The English Department for Education has stated that it would like all children to understand by the end of secondary school that 'all pornography presents a distorted picture of sexual behaviours, can damage the way people see themselves in relation to others and negatively affect how they behave towards sexual partners' (Hanson, 2020).

Research into the impact of pornography on the lives of our young people has found that it is does seem to increase the likelihood of 'at least some individuals behaving sexually coercively or aggressively' (Hanson, 2020). The same research also indicates that it may reduce the chance of people intervening in risky situations as 'positive bystanders' because they become used to watching violence and sexual material without acknowledging or allowing feelings of distress, confusion, shock or concern. According to Hanson (2020), free online pornography:

> often depicts violence, exploitation, humiliation and denigration, in most part towards women. For example, in a content analysis of 400 of the most popular free online pornography films, Klaassen and Peter (2015) found that 41% of professional videos depicted violence towards women (this figure dropped to 37% when films labelled 'amateur' were also included). The two most common forms of violence were spanking and gagging (inserting a penis very far into the mouth). (Hanson, 2020)

Therefore, research and working practice with young people suggests that sexual activity that is violent and exploitative has been normalized, leading to less sensitivity regarding mutual consent and mutual pleasure throughout the experience. That men are entitled to use women's bodies to gratify their sexual desires even while they are absent is far removed from the act of sex being a mutual expression of respect, love and genuine care for the other. The concept of intimacy seems to have come far away from emotional connection that naturally leads to physical connection. While sexual desire has seemed to separate from intimate emotional connection, the consequences seem to be a profound feeling of disconnection and loneliness, resulting in addictive needs to feel alive and connected and thus looking for sexual activity in easy-to-access ways.

Men and boys are the primary users of pornography (Flood, 2009; Boyle, 2010; Horvath *et al.*, 2013). In research in 2013, 'both young women and young men concluded that pornography not only eroticises men's dominance over women, sexualising sexism, but also that this influences their perceptions of their young female peers' (Coy *et al.*, 2013, p.45).

## Sexting and sexual harassment

Sexting has been defined as 'the creation and transmission of sexual images through social media and communication technology, usually with reference to young people' (Hanson, 2020). Research in England has concluded that sexting is part of young people's lives and is neither shocking nor surprising to them (Phippen, 2012). However, it is recognized that it can cause deep distress and many young people report shock, disgust, unwanted sexual experiences and communication with coercion that makes them feel powerless. Children need to be aware that they may feel scared, shocked and confused, and want to ask questions and seek reassurance and support from adults as they navigate this.

## The impact of sexual trauma

When a child is made to endure any sexually abusive experiences, they react instinctively to what feels like an overwhelming situation. For many, it will feel like a life and death situation, while others may at first feel terrified and awkward, but then overwhelmed and disgusted. Some may immediately feel shocked, numb, terrified and horrified. The child's survival instinct enables them to use clever subconscious mechanisms to survive what can feel unsurvivable. The child can immediately feel overwhelming terror and powerlessness, while realizing within seconds that they are completely stuck. Here are some examples of how adults tell their stories of childhood sexual abuse and describe themselves:

'I couldn't move. I was frozen and couldn't scream. I was just like a rag doll, with no breath, suffocated in the shock of what was happening.'

'I thought I was going to die. I didn't know what was happening. I left my body.'

'I screamed but the scream didn't seem to come out. It was like I was gasping. I couldn't move. I then tried to scrub everything off my body, but I never felt fully clean. I felt dirty.'

'It was a secret that I was told I had to keep, but it was also a secret that I kept from myself as the horror was too overwhelming. I didn't have words. I wanted it to go away. It took me 15 years until I broke the silence.'

'I left my body in a split second and watched from the ceiling. I could see a body being hurt and horrid stuff happening. I kind of knew it was me, but it didn't feel real.'

'I froze and had to remember to breathe. I still find that I feel frozen and my breathing feels like it can sometimes "catch".'

These words that describe how people felt when they were abused as children explain why the common suggestion for someone who has experienced this type of trauma to 'take time to talk about what has happened' or 'just tell us so we can help you?' doesn't work well and can add to the turmoil and confusion.

The child can be left with confusion, shame and terror of many different unfamiliar or familiar situations and people. It can take them time to process the layers of emotions, unconscious coping mechanisms, their thinking, all relationships and their relationship with their own body.

## Shame as a blanket that covers and hides them

The areas I cover in greater depth in *The Simple Guide to Understanding Shame in Children* (2018) are vital to facilitating recovery from sexual trauma because the child will almost always assume it is their fault that it happened and that is why they usually don't disclose it to anyone immediately. Shame causes them to keep the secret and then feel bad about themselves for 'letting it happen to them', despite somehow knowing that they were utterly powerless. It is the shame of what they saw, what they did or what they didn't say afterwards that can cripple them for years and decades. The other dilemma is the knowledge that sexual predators are aware that while the child will feel terror, powerlessness and overwhelm, they may simultaneously feel chosen, wanted and loved and it may have one element of feeling nice. If a child has previously felt rejected, neglected, overlooked or ugly, then they can sometimes enjoy the feeling of being chosen, which is confusing for them because they also hated everything about the abuse and felt that they may die.

Many children can eventually explore the level of shame that they felt about the experience. They realize that it hindered their sense of freedom and innocence and put a filter on how they view the world and how they fit in it. Shame makes people feel as if they don't fit in – they are bad; they are unwanted; they are broken; they are seen as a problem; things are probably their fault – and so they often try and hide or avoid any situation where they may experience further shame. One of the most important sentences to repeat to someone who has experienced sexual abuse is 'it was not your fault', because while they know that to be true, there can be a sense of wondering why it happened to them and what they did to cause the devastating impact of the terrifying experience. That sentence reduces shame and identifies them as a victim and the trauma as an injustice.

If you are reading this as an adult who was sexually abused as a child or as a young person, I want you to know that it was not your fault. You never should have been hurt in that way.

## Their body

Children who are sexually abused often have to dissociate in order to survive. They can dissociate or feel as if they are separated from their body in some way, so they don't feel the discomfort, pain, terror or overwhelming physical or emotional sensations. This is called depersonalization and is a common symptom of having been physically violated, but it leads to challenges with feeling their body in day-to-day life. They can struggle to know when they

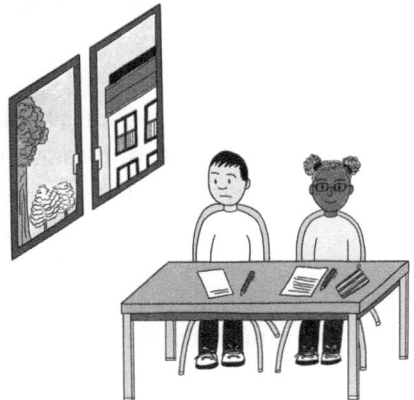

are hungry or full, thirsty or needing the toilet. They can sometimes notice that they have had an injury, but they don't notice the pain or bleeding. It is a coping mechanism that enabled the child to avoid having to be aware of body memories in their day-to-day life. It doesn't dissolve the memories because they are stored in their subconscious and can cause flashbacks and nightmares, seemingly out of nowhere. They can also avoid feeling revulsion about their body in their day-to-day life, although that too can be buried in the subconscious as a feeling that is now disconnected to any past experience.

A child who has experienced sexual abuse can have an avoidant relationship with their body where they want to pretend it is not there because it has done bad things and been in bad places, or they want to control their body so that they don't feel powerless again. This impacts their relationship with food, sport, their sexual development, medical or health challenges and relationships with all adults who they thought were there to protect them. They will need help to process the trauma and at the same time help their bodies process the shock, horror, pain and physical terror of what happened. Wieland (2011) explains how:

> the child's brain may need to be retaught (or for very early dissociation, taught) how to be aware of physical, emotional and cognitive responses. The child may need to be taught to see and recognize his or her body and body reactions as part of herself because it can feel so alien to them. (p.14)

## Symptoms that can develop due to sexual trauma

Sexual abuse can:

- change a person's breathing due to the shock and sudden intake of breath, and then they can often struggle to breathe in the physical panic
- change a person's view of their body and how they look after it
- change a person's understanding of sex, genitals and their sexuality
- make them feel as if they are dirty, disgusting, used and discarded
- cause anxiety, depression and self-loathing, self-hatred and rejection of themselves and of others

- cause an obsession with sex and a lack of appropriate boundaries with their own body
- cause them to subconsciously seek further abuse and mistreatment, sometimes to re-enact the feeling of abuse in order to try and process it
- cause exhaustion because of the weight of keeping such a secret
- cause anger and agitation towards anyone who makes them feel powerless
- cause them to experience depersonalization where they don't feel their body or an aspect of it, or derealization where they spend time in their own world to avoid the turmoil of the here and now
- cause them to feel numb and then use self-harm to help them know they are alive
- cause them to feel body pain in areas that were hurt, such as wrists, ankles, neck and genitals
- cause them to control or avoid other children so that they can avoid being powerlessness
- disturb the child's sleep, eating, toileting and overall health
- cause them to develop sexually addictive or avoidant behaviours.

## Their changed worldview

Sexual abuse also changes the child's view of the world and their day-to-day life. They may see the world as a dangerous place and think that they are responsible for awful things that happened to them when they felt so powerless. Sexual abuse can also involve payment and bribes, which can make a child feel guilty or have an ambivalent relationship with money or gifts.

Sadly, it is often a reality that 'experiences of emotional, physical, and/or sexual abuse create identities of being bad, deserving of harm or useful only for the satisfaction of adults' (Gomez-Perales, 2015, p.12). The route to recovery from sexual abuse is when they can experience positive, healing relationships with others who treat them with dignity and care for them and their body. When others help them to care for their body while they begin to realize, one layer at a time, that what happened to them was not their fault, they will then be able to slowly thank their body for surviving and keeping them alive. This enables them to begin to see good people in a world that has some abusers within it, and so their worldview can become more hope filled and less full of terror.

## Triggers

Children may be triggered by all the different aspects of the memory of the abuse but also by daily experiences such as washing, toileting, changing for sport, swimming with minimal clothing on, periods, genital discharge and going to places where they are not sure who will be present. They are unlikely to be able to explain that and will often not be aware that what they feel and are experiencing is a 'trigger' of a past experience. They may feel confused, terrified, avoidant and stupid that they are having what can seem like such a disproportionate reaction to a minor experience. They may dissociate and 'float' through the challenges with little awareness of what they are doing in order to numb the distress and turmoil that they feel inside.

'I was having a normal day, but someone grabbed my wrist in a game and I suddenly shouted, "No one touches that" and then ran away crying. A teacher found me frozen and staring while holding my knees in the corner of the school grounds, sitting on the grass. I hadn't noticed it was wet and when she came near me I shook. That freaked me out. I didn't know what was happening.' *Jane, aged 13*

## Speaking about it

When someone has been abused in this way, it can often take them a long time to say the words that describe what happened. When they hear their own voice saying what happened, it can cause psychological shock as they desperately wish they could 'un-say' the words and pretend it never happened. This is why denial can be easier in the short term and more natural than asking for help or telling others. The feeling of terror that they may be punished, hated, further abused or shamed can be overwhelming, and it can take time and support for them to trust that the adults who are helping them believe they didn't provoke this abuse, it wasn't their fault and they won't get into trouble. We then need to make sure we have plans to enable them to be safe and not have threats or actual further harm for speaking up about what happened.

## Disgust

The symptom of disgust is often not acknowledged as present in the aftermath of sexual trauma, where it is common for children to show symptoms of feeling sick or wanting to be sick if they think about what happened.

> Noses, mouths, and tongues will scrunch up often as a prelude to a memory. It is crucial to accept these signs and symptoms as a desire for the body to complete its defensive 'disgust responses' by exploring them with curiosity until they subside on their own. (Levine & Kline, 2017, p.257)

The response needs to be validated by the supporting adults and facilitated to be discharged with enough room to express it with emotional and somatic expression. Sometimes working with sensory materials such as slime and gunk can facilitate this feeling and can enable it to be processed with careful attunement, kindness, empathy and validation. The child may feel disgust about every aspect of having a body, from eating, breathing, their nose, fingernails, face and all the details that other children may not notice. They can become hypervigilant about not being disgusting or they may have to dissociate or numb so that they can still the internal feeling of self-disgust.

## Ideas to help a child recover from sexual trauma

The child will need help to do the following:

- Develop a positive relationship with their body, with work around who they are, what they can feel, what happens when they eat, move and why they need to wash, what functions are normal for the body, and many other aspects. This can be facilitated by both the parent or carer and the therapist.
- Release some of the emotions that they were unable to express during the abuse, such as anger, injustice, disgust, sadness,

shock, confusion. These can be expressed creatively with a creative therapist in a way that the child is comfortable with and prepared for.

- Explore themes such as dirty and clean; feeling nice and not feeling nice; control and powerlessness; frozen and stuck; ambivalence and loyalty; silence and silent screaming; secrets and shame; injustice and justice. This can be carefully led by a therapist, as some of these subjects are thoughts and issues that are unconscious due to the terror. Once they have been helped to the conscious by the therapist, then the child may choose to explore them with their other adults, or they may choose not to.
- Explore their coping mechanisms such as dissociation, both depersonalization and derealization, and their fight, flight or freeze reaction. This needs to be led by the therapist as it is an exploration of the unconscious.
- Explore their trauma symptoms, such as flashbacks, nightmares, startle response, body memories, addictive behaviours and other body trauma symptoms.
- Explore how they can begin to feel safe in different settings, such as changing for sport or swimming, going to a friend's house, sleepovers and other new settings and spaces.
- Cope with examinations of their genitals for medical reasons. These can be terrifying, and they will probably need additional support for that, even as they enter adulthood, with prostate checks or vaginal examinations such as smears.
- Learn to assess risk. The child may feel drawn to experiences of risk and feelings of danger because that can be associated with some attention, which, although terrifying, may also come with a feeling of being alive. They may now 'normalize' feelings of danger and feel more comfortable in that environment than in what others call 'safe'.
- Explore boundaries and what makes them feel unsafe and safe. Sexual trauma is a breach of personal boundaries that causes trauma that is deep and enduring. Levine and Kline (2017) offer clear instructions:

> Children, therefore, need to be protected by honouring their right to personal space, privacy, and to be in charge of their

own body. As different situations develop at various stages and ages, children need to know that they do not have to subject themselves to 'sloppy kisses', lap sitting, and other forms of unwanted attention to please the adults in their life. (p.245)

- Practise shouting 'no' loudly in role plays to help them experience the power of their voice and what a boundary means. They can explore their feelings when people are close to them physically and when they feel safe and when they don't. They need to explore those feelings they have when they feel 'weird' or 'funny' inside and don't know why. What could those feelings be saying? Could they be warning them that it is not safe?

We recognize that all humans tend to freeze when faced with terror and abuse, and yet sadly many can feel confused or shame about why they didn't kick, scream or shout because they don't understand the instinctive reaction of silence and stillness to avoid death. Children who have been abused previously could be even less able to shout or kick or run due to the freeze response being familiar and causing them to 'give in' to abuse because fighting or shouting won't work. The pre-used coping mechanism of freeze or dissociation can instinctively be activated by a minor attempt at violation, and therefore we need to work hard to help these children develop strong reactions to danger so that they are equipped more to avoid further abuse.

## Therapeutic story books that explore prevention and disclosure of sexual abuse

There are some good books that help children to listen and reflect on someone else's story, which feels far less invasive and painful. Here are a few:

- *Your Body Belongs to You* by Cornelia Spelman (1997). Albert Whitman & Company. (This book also helps the child begin to take ownership over their own body so that they feel empowered to say 'No – my body belongs to me'.)
- *Some Secrets Should Never Be Kept* by Janeen Sanders (2011). Upload Publishing.

## Disclosures

If a child discloses new information or important memories about sexual abuse that occurred, it is vital that the appropriate professionals are informed. It is essential that the words of the child are written down as they were said, with no words added. The child may want to help you with that, or they may not. It is important to be kind, empathetic and warm as they speak, and to remain non-judgemental and unemotional, but not casual and uncaring, so that the child feels supported and heard. If the child is in danger, the police need to be told immediately. The child must be assured that you care, and they won't get into trouble. They need to be told that you must work with the professionals who are there to make sure children can be safe and protected. The social care child protection team or the police child investigation team who are on duty need to be contacted and they will guide the process of any involvement of the criminal justice system.

## Prevention of further abuse

The best way to help children prevent further abuse is to help them process the abuse so that they no longer think it was their fault. When they can see that they were powerless and terrified, and it was therefore a serious crime and injustice against them, and that they now have some new methods to use to get help quickly, they can begin to feel the weight of worry lessen. They need to thank and acknowledge their survival and coping mechanisms and notice when they are using them, in the hope they decrease as they begin to feel safer.

To empower them to stop further abuse, they may like to take up classes in self-defence or work on building strong muscles, so they feel able to kick or punch. They may want to develop an alert or safe word so that they can always ask for help in a less awkward way on a phone call with others listening or in a text that may be viewed.

'If someone had asked me if I was abused at any time before I was 16, I would have said no. Once two lovely women did and I laughed. Inside my head I did wonder though what they meant and I couldn't stop crying. It took me another four years to finally tell one person and another ten years to really believe it. The abuse had been a part of my life since I was 4.' *Susan, aged 32*

## Conclusion

Trauma recovery is possible, even for the person who has experienced severe and organized sexual abuse. The memories can become less potent and lose their grip on the person's reactions, relationships and anxiety. Processing this trauma is beyond painful at the start, and sometimes the acknowledgement of it happening at all can take years, but once the memories have begun to be accepted and the story unfolds, it can make sense of other coping mechanism and fears, which can bring a sense of hope. To walk through the darkness of the reality of an abuser's evil intent can be horrific, and the journey needs to be planned, with enough supporters, enough methods of bringing calm and beauty, and enough stories of others who have made it through the depths of pain to the other side where hope is strong and peace is a reality.

# CHAPTER 19

# Physical Abuse

Physical abuse causes devastation to a child, especially when the adult hurting the child is the person who is meant to protect and care for them. This violation can cause attachment trauma, which then impacts their other relationships because of the anxiety around trusting people. The child can be left with pain, injury or marks on their skin that they try and hide to protect their abusers, due to the shame that they feel about it happening to them.

Because all children are developmentally appropriate in their ego-centricity in order to survive life and get their needs met, they can usually assume that they are bad rather than the abuser is bad. While this may make no logical sense to many adults, it is the nature of abuse, and so a child often remains silent about harm that their adult may cause to them. They have an instinctive internal drive to protect and defend their adult, and a terror of what may happen if they ever told the truth of the abuse, and so if a teacher or supporter asks a child if they have been harmed, it is common for a child to deny it.

Physical abuse can be described as:

- hitting the child in any way, including with objects
- slapping, punching, kicking, shaking or throwing them
- trying to suffocate them or stop them breathing
- pushing them into water or attempting to drown them
- poisoning or burning them
- biting or scratching them
- controlling their food intake so they are hungry
- breaking their bones.

## Attachment trauma

The confusion and chaos that physical abuse causes can lead to long-term relational challenges, where trust is complex and therefore emotional closeness can feel unsafe. When a child has trusted an adult who has then hurt them, it can leave them unsure of who to trust, if anyone, and they can withdraw and become independent, self-sufficient, 'loners', avoidant of emotional intimacy or sharing themselves in a way where they could get rejected or further hurt. There is further reading about attachment trauma in my book *The Simple Guide to Attachment Difficulties* (2019); for a child with attachment trauma and showing signs of dissociation, you may find it helpful to carry out some further background reading in *The Simple Guide to Complex Trauma and Dissociation* (2000).

The shock of the physical abuse can cause children to live their whole lives either avoidant of further harm by being people pleasers and compliant or by finding power and strength so that others may feel too threatened to attempt to harm them. Or they can become numb, be in denial, dissociative and feel as if they are living life on one level rather than with a full force of energy and awareness of where they fit into the world and those around them. Or they can become angry, agitated, aggressive and ready to defend themselves at the slightest hint of attack.

'She was mad and held her hand over my face so I could hardly breathe. I almost died but she pushed my head out of the window to breathe while telling me to be quiet, so the neighbours didn't hear. My eyes became blood shot, so I had to miss school. I think I first told someone about that around 20 years later.' *Jeremy, aged 30, looking back at being aged 17*

## Psychological shock

When a child is used to being cared for and stroked, cuddled, rocked or carried, they can go into what is called psychological shock when the same adult then hurts them. They can immediately become pale and silent, their breathing becomes shallow, they can look blank, feel sick or become twitchy or clingy, or they may cry. They may lose the usual energy that a child has when they are healthy, and they may become less bouncy, less playful and slower in their movements. Or they may become angry and aggressive, and can even hit or hurt other children, sometimes to almost 'see what happens', which can help them explore what has happened to them in a more subconscious way.

If a child has not known consistent, kind, caring touch and gentle soothing movements, then they may be less shocked but may continue to show the above symptoms in a more continual activated freeze response.

## Bullying

Often a child is bullied with a combination of physical attack and verbal aggression. When a child is bullied, they can experience:

- being hit, scratched, punched or hurt physically
- being picked on and teased
- being mocked for something they did, said, wore or suggested
- being purposefully set up to look as if they did something they didn't, so they are 'told off'
- having their property taken, broken, hidden, thrown around or shown to others
- being made to feel or be isolated, lonely, shamed or that something is wrong with them
- being lied about so that they get into trouble while others laugh
- having others manipulate or twist facts to tease them
- having others try to align people against them.

Vital research by Wolke and Lereya (2015) exploring the long-term effects of bullying provides this definition:

> Bullying is the systematic abuse of power and is defined as aggressive behaviour or intentional harm-doing by peers that is carried out repeatedly and involves an imbalance of power. Being bullied is still often wrongly considered as a 'normal rite of passage'.

They found the alarming statistics of children and young people who have experienced bullying:

One in three children report having been bullied at some point in their lives, and 10–14% experience chronic bullying lasting for more than 6 months. Between 2% and 5% are bullies and a similar number are bully/victims in childhood/adolescence. Rates of cyberbullying are substantially lower at around 4.5% for victims and 2.8% for perpetrators (bullies and bully/victims), with up to 90% of the cyber-bullying victims also being traditionally (face to face) bullied. Being bullied by peers is the most frequent form of abuse encountered by children, much higher than abuse by parents or other adult perpetrators. (Wolke & Lereya, 2015)

## Symptoms that can develop due to physical abuse

- Hypervigilance – they may need to sit with their back to the wall or in a place where no one can come up from behind them to hurt them.
- Being twitchy and agitated as they try and prepare themselves for physical harm.
- Having bruises, marks or wounds that they try and avoid letting people see, and stopping wearing certain clothes, or having additional clothes on to hide them.
- Lying about how they got the wounds to protect the adult.
- Showing anxiety about going to the place where they get hurt, and showing signs of distress.
- Dissociating from their body and not noticing if they are hungry, thirsty or need the toilet or if they fall over and cut themselves. They may be spoken of as 'having a high pain tolerance'.
- Stopping eye contact with people, trying to seem invisible so that they don't attract further abuse.
- Showing disproportionate emotional expression for minor stimuli because they are living in a state of agitation.
- Being dissociative and floating around, hardly connecting with others and seeming to be relaxed and avoidant of conflict.
- Becoming the class clown and making fun of everything to hide how sad they are.
- Hitting or kicking another person and being known for being

aggressive because they don't know you aren't meant to be, as that is what they have experienced.

## Trauma recovery from physical abuse

The trauma recovery pathway for a child who has been physically abused or bullied includes support from adults in processing the shock, turmoil, shame and confusion of what happened.

The child will need to try and make sense of what happened and also be prepared to defend themselves against further physical assault so that they feel less powerless and vulnerable and more prepared and equipped.

They need to understand the normal, automatic reactions that occur physically in an experience where they feel terrified. They need to be able to explore why they may not have screamed, why they may not have told someone immediately, their fear of getting the other person into trouble, their worry that no one can stop it happening and the feelings of intense shame and turmoil that it did happen to them.

They may withdraw from other relationships while they feel that their trust was breached, and they may dissociate from their body so that they can avoid any body memories coming back to shock them and remind them of what happened.

They may have an ambivalent relationship with their body and may need to learn to look after it and care for it.

The journey of trauma recovery from physical abuse follows a similar path as someone who has experienced other traumas that impact their body, mind, emotions, relationships and subconscious (see Sections 1 and 2) because they had to develop coping mechanisms and defence mechanisms to survive what felt life threatening to them. Recovery needs to be facilitated for all those areas impacted.

If it is a peer abuse situation, then the relationship with the school or organization where the bullying is happening is vital, as they need to be aware of the situation and should offer strategies and support for the child.

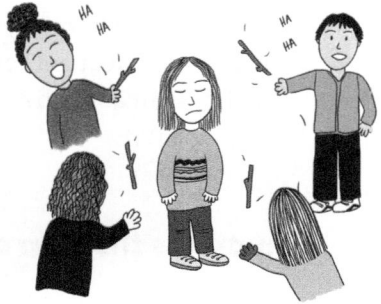

If it is interpersonal trauma, because the child has been physically abused by the adult(s) who should be the main caregiver, then the first matter for attention is the child's current physical safety. After that safeguarding process with social care, the parent will need some support, and the child will need space and time to process their internal confusion and attachment conflict. Following on from this immediate support, the child will also need to be able to build some therapeutic relationships with other safe adults who they can learn to trust.

## The primary themes to explore for recovery

The primary themes that need exploring when physical abuse has been experienced are usually powerlessness, terror, overwhelm, betrayal, shock, anger and relational confusion around trust and safety.

## Conclusion

Physical abuse does not just impact the physical body of the child; it impacts their perception of the world, their relationships, their self-esteem, their emotional regulation and their identity. They can either become quiet and withdrawn to avoid further conflict and pain or they may take up more space and be loud and aggressive so they can feel power over others because of the powerlessness that they feel when they are abused. They can recover, but first need help to have the physical abuse stop so that they can slowly begin to explore feeling safe in their body and emotions, before they can then process the feelings of terror, powerlessness and overwhelm.

# CHAPTER 20

# Emotional or Psychological Abuse

Emotional or psychological abuse can be more difficult to notice because there are no visible scars or wounds. Often a child who is being emotionally abused is living in a constant state of terror of others, which causes them to avoid the attention of other adults due to fear of further harm. The lack of physical signs of their suffering can exacerbate the feeling of confusion and shame, because the other adults around them are often unaware of the turmoil that the child is experiencing. As with children experiencing other abuses, they are rarely able to put into words what they feel, what is happening and what they need from others, because of the depth of turmoil, confusion, shock, terror and loyalty to the adults who they depend on for food, drink and a bed. What they need is for one or more adults to invest time into connecting with them and offering them opportunities to be known, seen and cared for and then they can begin to explore what a safe relationship feels like. Over time, the child may be able to offer hints or small elements of stories that can begin to paint the picture of what turmoil they are experiencing.

Iram Rizvi and Najam researched the prevalence of psychological abuse and the longer-term impact on the child's development and found that it is a significant worldwide problem.

Psychological abuse (PA) is an under recognized and under reported phenomena especially in the adolescents by their own parents. It has been described as the most challenging as well as the most prevalent form of child abuse. PA is rather difficult to define and assess compared to physical abuse and may be described as, verbal abuse, harsh nonphysical punishments, or threats of abuse. It describes a repeated pattern of adult-to-child behaviour (usually a parent) that makes the child feel worthless, flawed, unloved, unwanted, endangered, or only of value in meeting another's needs. (Iram Rizvi & Najam, 2014)

They evidenced that the impact of a child experiencing this kind of abuse is a wide range of symptoms such as:

depression; anxiety, low-self-esteem, and eating disorders. In turn, these problems are associated with physical health problems, including over-all poor physical health, increased risk of heart disease, self-injurious behaviours. This type of abuse can be extremely destructive and has been associated with a range of adverse child outcomes including emotional maladjustment, depression, poor self-esteem, conduct problems, aggression, inability to trust, and underachievement.

A child can recover from the impact of psychological abuse, but it can be difficult for them to ask for the help they need because many are terrified of any disclosure that may increase the harm and terror before any justice can be established.

## The foundation of safety and stability

As has been explored in this book, the foundation that needs to be built for trauma recovery is one of safety and stability, where the child feels able to explore the feeling of being safe, emotionally, psychologically and physically. The challenge in this trauma experience is that the child is limited in how much they can recover while they are still living in the environment of abuse, and as such the transition to a home that can become safe and stable needs to be the main priority. While the child is still living in the chaos of psychological abuse, they would benefit from supportive, therapeutic adults who enable them to explore their feelings and their symptoms of distress and help them feel less alone and stuck. These relationships will contribute to the process of building that foundation, but until they are no longer living in that environment, they will not be able to process the full trauma of it because they still need their coping mechanisms to survive what could happen to them and what they still have to witness and be submerged within.

## Domestic violence or abuse

Domestic violence is a complex trauma experience that can vary in detail, but the main elements are of a child living in a home where there is fighting, emotional and/or physical abuse, manipulation and/or control and a lack of calm and healthy relationships that enable a child to feel safe and secure. Children naturally 'soak up' the atmosphere of their home, and as they witness and sense the complexities of the relationships, they can feel terrified and powerless when they are enfolded in an abusive home. Sadly, the impact on the child when there is violence at home 'has powerful effects on brains and nervous systems (McTavish *et al.*, 2016), often worse than being the recipient of violence oneself (Teicher & Samson 2016)' (Music, 2019, p.29).

It needs to be acknowledged that it is not easy for the adult victim of domestic abuse or violence, and they can feel trapped and terrified and be confused about how to get support for what is happening. The domestic abuse perpetrator is usually able to manipulate the victim in a way that confuses them, often by fluctuating between being flattering and generous, maybe even with promises of holidays or presents, to abusing, controlling or mocking them. The power dynamic can cause such confusion that the adult victim may take some time to recognize the signs of abuse and seek help, but then the process of leaving the relationship can be terrifying, confusing and overwhelming. The perpetrator can use the ownership of the home, money, gifts or the children to manipulate the victim, and therefore seeking help can take great courage, wisdom and support.

The NSPCC (2024) describes domestic abuse as:

> Domestic abuse is any type of controlling, bullying, threatening or violent behaviour between people who are or have been in a relationship. It can also happen between adults related to one another. It can seriously harm children and young people, and experiencing domestic abuse is child abuse.
>
> It's important to remember that domestic abuse:

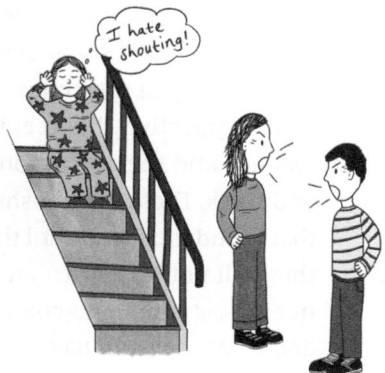

- can happen inside and outside the home
- can happen over the phone, on the internet and on social net-working sites.
- can happen in any relationship and can continue even after the relationship has ended.
- both men and women can be abused or abusers.

Domestic abuse can be emotional, physical, sexual, economic, coercive or psychological, such as:

- kicking, hitting, punching, cutting or throwing objects
- rape (including in a relationship)
- controlling someone's finances by withholding money or stop-ping someone earning
- controlling behaviour, like telling someone where they can go and what they can wear
- not letting someone leave the house
- reading emails, text messages or letters
- threatening to kill someone or harm them
- threatening to another family member or pet. (NSPCC, 2024)

Children are harmed when they grow up in this environment, and the symptoms of distress are described and explored in Sections 1 and 2 of this book. Research has shown that 'parent reports in daily home diaries revealed that a high percentage of children exhibited fear, flight (e.g., left the room), fight (e.g., took sides), and social de-escalation (e.g., tried to make peace) behaviors in response to interparental conflict' (Davies & Martin, 2008).

The child may grow up hearing the shouting or violence, their own food or access to their home being restricted, their loved one feeling distressed or being hurt, finding broken furniture or parts of the home, or living in silent and scary atmospheres that make them feel unsafe. While they may not feel like the main victim of the abuse, they sadly do become victims of the traumatic experience, and it can impact their behaviour, body, emotions, thinking, relationships and subconscious. They need support to be able to have the experience validated as ter-rifying, where they felt powerless and overwhelmed, and be helped to explore what they feel like and what they can do to keep themselves safe. The trauma recovery journey for all children who are traumatized can be followed in Sections 1 and 2.

> 'I thought it was my mum that had the issues because she was the one who was always shouting. Then I realized my dad was the issue and she was protecting us. It was awful and I always hoped they would just shut up.' *Ryan, aged 12*

## Coercive control

This can be an element of a domestic abusive home, or it can be that one of the adults in the child's world is using coercive control to wield power over another person in the family or the child. Often children who grow up in a home where coercive control is present can show behaviours that are more submissive, compliant and people pleasing, because they live with such terror that things could become even worse than they currently are. Within coercive control is the method of terrifying the child that they are powerless, and the adult has all the power, and therefore the child often becomes silent and submissive. When a child grows up in this home setting, they can show symptoms of distress, which on the Window of Tolerance includes both the hyper-arousal behaviours and the hypoarousal behaviours (see Chapter 2), although they usually present as more hypoaroused due to feeling as if their lives are threatened all the time.

This is the definition of coercive control from the Crown Prosecution Service (2023):

Section 76 Serious Crime Act 2015 (SCA 2015) created the offence of controlling or coercive behaviour in an intimate or family relationship (CCB).

Relevant behaviour of the suspect can include:

- isolating a person from their friends and family
- depriving them of their basic needs
- monitoring their time
- monitoring a person via online communication tools or using spyware
- using digital systems such as smart devices or social media to

coerce, control, or upset the victim including posting triggering material

- taking control over aspects of their everyday life, such as where they can go, who they can see, what to wear and when they can sleep – this can be intertwined with the suspect saying it is in their best interests, and 'rewarding' 'good behaviour' e.g. with gifts
- depriving them of access to support services, such as specialist support or medical services
- repeatedly putting them down such as telling them they are worthless
- enforcing rules and activity which humiliate, degrade or dehumanize the victim
- forcing the victim to take part in criminal activity such as shoplifting, neglect or abuse of children to encourage self-blame and prevent disclosure to authorities
- economic abuse including coerced debt, controlling spending/bank accounts/investments/mortgages/benefit payments
- controlling the ability to go to school or place of study
- taking wages, benefits or allowances
- threatening to hurt or kill
- threatening to harm a child
- threatening to reveal or publish private information
- threatening to hurt or physically harming a family pet
- assault
- physical intimidation e.g. blocking doors, clenching or shaking fists
- criminal damage (such as destruction of household goods)
- preventing a person from having access to transport or from working
- preventing a person from learning or using a language or making friends outside of their ethnic or cultural background
- family 'dishonour'
- reputational damage
- sexual assault or threats of sexual assault
- reproductive coercion, including restricting a victim's access to birth control, refusing to use a birth control method, forced pregnancy, forcing a victim to get an abortion, to undergo in

vitro fertilization (IVF) or other procedure, or denying access to such a procedure
- using substances such as alcohol or drugs to control a victim through dependency, or controlling their access to substances
- disclosure of sexual orientation
- disclosure of HIV status or other medical condition without consent
- limiting access to family, friends and finances
- withholding and/or destruction of the victim's immigration documents, e.g. passports and visas
- threatening to place the victim in an institution against the victim's will, e.g. care home, supported living facility, mental health facility, etc (particularly for disabled or elderly victims).

## Living through the child

Some parents who may have themselves been traumatized as a child can fail to keep the boundaries of the role of parent and instead 'live through their child' by experiencing elements of childhood that they felt they were robbed of as they watch their child or do the activity with them. The adult can then become an 'onlooker', which can hinder the child's freedom due to the nature of the 'watching' or can lead the child to feel that they don't have an adult caregiver but instead a traumatized child in an adult body who is seeking friendship with them. Sometimes the parent will believe that their 'watching' is because they are being attentive and emotionally present, but the child's experience of it is being trapped and used.

'My mum has been struggling with her mental health and she is the only parent watching us at ballet. I can't really dance how I would like as I feel stared at and I know she is watching me to process some of her stuff.' *Sindy, aged 12*

## Bullying

Bullying can be either physical, emotional or sexual or a combination of these abuses. It can happen both in person and also online and can cause significant distress, despair and other trauma symptoms to develop due to the child trying to survive that which feels terrifying and where they often feel shame for being picked on. Emotional, verbal or psychological abuse is explored in Chapter 19 on physical abuse.

When it is online, the child can struggle to feel as if they will ever get away from the source of pain and distress, and it can seem invasive and unrelenting. While physical abuse can sometimes have bruises, wounds and eventually scars that can tell the story of what happened and sometimes elicit empathy, sadly emotional abuse, cyber stalking and harassment can be seen as less destructive. Empathy and kindness are often less available for those who experience these less publicly witnessed traumatic experiences, which increases loneliness, shame and confusion as the child wonders if they are at fault. This can lead to the child self-harming or causing physical injury to elicit the kind of care that those who are physically unwell seem to be able to access. It can also lead to them withdrawing and avoiding all human interaction due to the assumption that they will become further hurt.

More on bullying can be found in Chapter 19, and more on sexting can be found in Chapter 18.

## Symptoms that can develop due to emotional or psychological abuse

The child may:

- avoid conflict, failure or further rejection by making choices that limit the possibility – this often looks as if they are being 'non-engaging' when they are actually avoiding further pain
- avoid all relationships, even those with people who seem to care, in case they suddenly change and become abusive
- show signs of being dissociative and not present in all activities, which can look as if they are daydreaming or not interested
- be a 'loner' and not have many friends because they don't want to have friends around at their home
- have an over-exaggerated reaction to minor conflict due to the subconscious or conscious assumption that the conflict will escalate into a terrifying experience
- be unfamiliar with adults who say sorry or who are able to reflect on mistakes they have made

- have expensive presents that seem out of context, or have expensive day trips to amazing places because they are being bribed to not tell people what is going on at home
- struggle to learn and reflect and instead be interruptive, mess around or avoid learning in any way they can as they struggle to concentrate on the here and now due to the wiring of their brain that stays alert for danger.

## Resources to help

Here is a therapeutic story book that can help:

- *The Boy Who Built a Wall Around Himself* by Ali Redford (2015). Jessica Kingsley Publishers.

## Conclusion

Emotional or psychological abuse can be devastating and cause the child to feel trapped in a situation that often others can't see, which they may find difficult to put into words. The consequential lack of empathy and compassion for those experiencing this trauma can hinder the recovery process and cause them to survive rather than make any attempt to 'confront or escape'. To confront their abuser can feel life threatening, and yet to stay within the environment or relationships that are emotionally abusive can also be life threatening. The feeling of being trapped can escalate the trauma symptoms and the child may resign themselves to a life of turmoil and emotional pain. The child needs emotional support and gentle care to be able to eventually speak about how they feel.

# CHAPTER 21

# Medical Trauma

When a child becomes seriously unwell with life-altering challenges that require medical intervention and may involve hospitals or long-term treatment, they can become traumatized. The whole family may also be impacted by the experience due to the change of focus in the family diary, which is now centred on medical visits and checks. The siblings may feel as if they are less important or valued because they have less attention or time spent on them, and the child who is unwell may feel guilty for changing the family routines and seeing the impact on others.

Arguably, the primary turmoil and impact of a period of time spent having medical treatment can be that the child often has to undergo treatments that save their life but make them feel as if the adult helper is abusing them or hurting them, and they feel powerless and terrified because they don't understand what is happening. This can be deeply distressing for all involved, but the child can be left confused about adults and why they do this while saying 'It's going to make you better'.

'Beyond the cure for childhood cancer…lie so many children whose mental health has been damaged so deeply that it affects all areas of their life… It is so sad. It is so hard to rationalize our gratitude for life, with the heartache of the scars left behind.' *Lizzie, mum who supported her young child through cancer treatment*

## The impact on the child

Sometimes hospital visits can be traumatizing for children 'because they lack control of their environment. This sense of helplessness, coupled with fear and pain can cause children to feel powerless in healthcare settings' (Lerwick, 2016). The child may experience and need to spend time exploring all the symptoms described in Sections 1 and 2 of this book, along with more specific symptoms and struggles such as:

- their ability to trust adults who have power – they may be terrified, may panic and may need more reassurance of what the adult is doing, why they are doing it and what would happen if they didn't do it (with age-appropriate language)
- why sometimes things have to hurt more before they get better – like childbirth or sometimes being sick if you have eaten something bad
- why they can be nervous around adults who aren't consistent in their behaviours
- consent and why some adults didn't stop when they wanted them to – how in other settings that would be wrong, but in this one the adults needed to overrule their opinion to save their life
- feeling heard and making choices – how adults need to listen to a child and value their opinion and thoughts, but there are rare occasions when the best thing they can do is to help the child stay alive.

## Validation

The first element of recovery from medical trauma is to acknowledge the confusion and turmoil that the child experiences and help them feel validated as they try and express the terror and powerlessness. It is important to give them time to explore this as it can be felt as psychological shock that causes the feelings and bodily sensations to be pushed down into the subconscious so that they can survive the short term. When any big emotions or body sensations are pushed away from consciousness, they can become like a volcano and seem to rumble and sometimes to erupt unless space is made to explore them and validate them with someone who shows authentic empathy, kindness and compassion without a hint of pity.

## Preparation for a child starting long-term medical support

While some medical interventions are emergencies and the atmosphere is filled with a dreadful feeling of life and death, others are planned, giving the parents opportunity to prepare the child as much as possible.

There is some interesting research into children's anxiety about being in hospital for treatment and these recognize that:

It is important that preparatory procedures and preadmission pro-grammes are made available for children. Nurses should promote a safe and supportive environment to help reduce children's anxieties, increase their understanding and facilitate overall coping. Helping children to express their fears and concerns and responding to those concerns is essential for successful outcomes. Parents play a significant role in reassuring their children and providing security and normality. Therefore, nurses should involve parents in the delivery of information so that they can help relieve children's anxieties. (Coyne & Conlan, 2007)

The child will need some routine and 'normality' and as much contact with their loved ones as possible. Play is vital and any opportunities or energy for play and creative expression can enable the child to process some of the big feelings of pain, turmoil, worry, confusion and sadness.

Here are some things that can help, which need to be reflected on so that the language used is age appropriate and doesn't unnecessarily cause increased fear for the child:

- Talking though what may happen and why, and who is going to be helping.
- Helping them explore what they may need to take with them which could help them feel more comfortable, less scared and more empowered.
- Discussing details such as what they can eat, where the toilets and toys will be, what they can do afterwards and the possible time restrictions on that, what medications they will need to take, what the pain may feel like and when it may be better.
- Showing them the different elements of their treatment, such as pictures of the tubes, the plaster and the children's ward, and allowing them to ask questions. It is important not to show them

anything that may further distress them, such any operating tools, scary-looking rooms, or any details of what may need to be done.

## Resources to help

It can be helpful to read age-appropriate therapeutic story books about others who have had to go to hospital, so that they can think through the details and be reassured that others have experienced it and can talk about it.

- *The Secret C: Straight Talking About Cancer* by Julie Stokes (2009). Winston's Wish (second revised edition).
- *Alice's Wonderful Hospital Adventure* by Tony Densely & Niki Palmer (2019). Westminster Designs.
- *Harry Goes to Hospital* by Howard Bennett (2008). Magination Press.

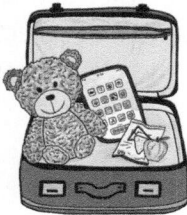

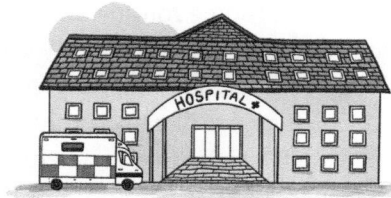

## Helping them tell others what happened

While some children may wish it had never happened and therefore never mention it again, others may need to be heard and they may need to tell their story. It can be therapeutic to help the child begin to work out a comfortable way to communicate what they have been enduring and why. They may prefer to do this in one sitting or over many weeks; in picture or art form or as a journal or photos. This ability to tell their story enables them to feel less isolated and more connected, and to reflect on what they want to share and what feels personal and too vulnerable to share.

Some children may not want to do this straight after a difficult period of time having treatment, but they may want to return to it after a while to help them discharge some of the turmoil, muddle and overwhelm, and they may need to ask questions to gain clarity on some aspects of their treatment. If they have a teacher, mentor, therapist or relative with whom they can share that book, poster, picture, journal, photo album or film of what they went through, this enables them to experience more validation and care, which helps them feel more supported and less confused or distressed about their experience.

## Conclusion

Children who have experienced life-saving medical care are caught in the dilemma of being grateful to be alive and yet often having a nagging sense of grief over things that they lost and a confusion about the process they had to endure. As they get older, they can often look back at the confusion they felt when they were little as they tried to understand that the adults who were saving their life felt like abusers, while the loving parent looked on in turmoil as they seemed to endorse the painful experience. This experience takes time to process and make sense of, and they can need space to grieve the loss of innocence about life and death, explore the themes of pain and powerlessness and what health and restoration feel like to them. Recovery is possible as the confusing threads of memories become less muddled and the emotions are felt, acknowledged and validated.

# CHAPTER 22

# Organizational Trauma

Trauma that impacts a child and their family due to an organization or 'system' rather than a person is sometimes called organizational trauma. When an organization is not trauma informed, it can cause children to feel further traumatized because they are not aware of the life-shattering impact that trauma can have on the lives of humans and what the symptoms are of that experience. The experience can be confusing as the child and family can experience powerlessness if there seems to be no way of moving forward and so many systems that don't listen or understand the needs of an individual. This can feel exhausting and can slowly cause the adult and the child to lose hope, and therefore other symptoms of distress to increase.

## Poverty

It is frustrating when we live in a world where there is enough food, but somehow it is not distributed equitably. Long-term poverty can impact a child's self-esteem, their health and their ability to learn and sustain friendships. It can cause shame to be deeply felt, and the child may want to pretend they have everything that their friends have because they may feel awkward to admit that they can't afford it. They may begin to think they are different, they don't fit in and they are 'less than' other children who seem to have the latest toys and enough healthy food.

When a family is facing poverty and feels shame about it, the adults may make sacrifices to give their children what they need, but then they may struggle with their own mental health issues due to the continual stress, disappointment and feelings of despair.

Poverty can cause the child to be hungry and that can stop them being able to learn easily. It may impact their clothes or toys and the child can feel left out of games where children show each other the latest item they have which is the current trend.

The child may:

- be tired due to sleeping conditions or lack of healthy food
- be angry due to feelings of injustice
- lie about what they own or where they live because the truth is too painful to be honest about
- steal food, money or other things to keep up with their friends
- feel left out, be a 'loner' and be withdrawn or quiet
- spend a lot of time online and then seem to struggle to stay in the here and now.

They may need:

- food that is consistent, and the ability to make some choices around food
- time to express the injustice of poverty
- an adult who will enable them to be heard and seen
- an adult who will help them begin to feel accepted so they can develop peer relationships
- the ability to reflect on what they want to do in their future and how they can achieve that so that they can feel reassured that poverty won't be a lifelong challenge.

## School systems

While there needs to be significant gratitude that people enter the profession of teaching to invest in the next generation, there can be challenges for them and the children within such an extraordinary organization that used to only focus on teaching but is now often the centre of social support for a geographical area, without additional finance to facilitate that resource. This incredible role within our communities is one that can often be expected by the parents and carers but not financed by the government or part of the mandate to 'educate children'. School leaders and

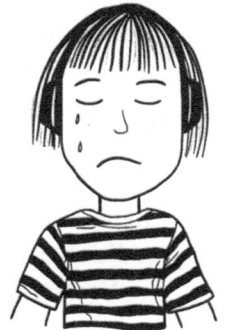

staff are often navigating demand for help with practical matters that is increasingly hard to fulfil, while other adults can forget that the school is trying to help practically in an area which is not their responsibility.

The changing role of schools within communities, alongside the pressure to evidence academic achievement, can become a toxic mix of stress, pressure and testing, without the financial resources to meet the increasingly diverse needs of the children who have survived significant national stressors. Traumatized children have differing needs and can need more relational support than is possible, despite many excellent school leaders, and while most children still thrive in the settings, some can struggle. When schools are able to offer this additional support, it does change the lives of those who would otherwise often end up feeling further abandoned by adults due to their unmet needs.

'When I changed schools, it changed everything. Here they trust me to go to the loo when I need it and let me drink if I need to and so I can concentrate on work stuff now.' *Carly, aged 13*

The lack of a trauma-informed approach within a school system can create a culture where authoritarian, frightening adults seem to dictate and rule the environment, using shame and punishment as ways to control behaviour. This approach causes shame and fear to escalate and that can cripple creativity, play, imagination and natural developmental curiosity. Children who are our future creatives, where they will be producing plays, films, music, dance, design and other parts of a rich community, can struggle within such atmospheres and become anxious and muddled. They can thrive when their specific skills are enabled to flourish and they are given support to get through the other aspects of their education.

The celebration of 100% attendance is not trauma informed because it immediately stops those who have medical issues or other challenges from being able to receive that affirmation and causes them to feel less a part of the community than others without these additional stresses.

Many schools are changing the lives of traumatized children, creating new systems and instilling new approaches that bring additional support and emotional safety to those who are finding life challenging.

The child may:

- want to avoid school because of fear of being shamed, failure or being misunderstood
- withdraw and avoid other people so that they can minimalize the need to try to explain what they are feeling and the vulnerability of that
- express self-rejection, self-hatred, insecurity, confusion or sadness about who they are
- lose confidence in social settings and begin to dread them or avoid them
- become agitated, on edge or anxious.

They may need:

- understanding from the adults around them
- reassurance that they are important, their voice matters and they are worthy of care.
- hope that they can find a setting where they can build positive relationships with peers and adults who can help them
- an adult to lead them through the suggested activities in Section 2 around emotions, relationships and the mind until they feel less overwhelmed and more able to speak about what is making them afraid and what they may need to move forward
- other spaces and places to experience peer friendships where they feel safe and accepted.

## Racism and cultural trauma

For a child or young person to live their life with a constant sense that they are perceived from a prejudiced lens can lead them to develop defensive mechanisms and coping mechanisms to survive that experience of trauma. Research has evidenced that for some people their experience can lead to a level of turmoil and distress where they develop symptoms of complex trauma:

Although complex trauma differs from racial trauma in its origin, the consistency of racist victimization beyond childhood, and the internalized racism associated with it, strong similarities exist. Similar to complex trauma, racial trauma surrounds the victims' life course and engenders consequences on their physical and mental health, behavior, cognition, relationships with others, self-concept, and social and economic life. (Cénat, 2023)

Until recently, there was little discourse on this trauma, which led to further shame and confusion regarding the experience. There are now excellent resources and further reading to equip professionals and families with knowledge of the specifics of how to facilitate recovery. We need to work hard to make sure that our cultures and teams are not racist, and that requires some attention to our subconscious experiences that shape our view of humanity.

Taking time to listen to those who may have experienced racism is vital, and then we need to move that into conversations that can implement change or challenge any processes around an adult's ability to encourage or ignore, champion or overlook, invest in or avoid children who may look different to them. Listening and being authentically committed to every person having the ability to be heard, seen, counted and valued is a foundational element of a trauma-informed system. It is vital that a child is valued, championed and listened to, so that they grow up knowing that they can achieve what they want to and that their voice matters.

Those who are seeking asylum or safety in our communities also need to be seen and heard as those who are often caught between wanting to stay where they felt at home but recognizing that the risk of danger was too high. They need support emotionally and practically to find their place in a community, where others can respect their courageous journey and learn about other parts of the world from a place of curiosity and compassion.

The child may:

- feel misunderstood and judged
- feel left out and isolated
- feel confused or shocked about the world they live in
- feel sad or depressed about the injustice of racism and prejudice
- feel anxious about what violence, bullying or hate crime they may experience

- struggle with good self-esteem and hope for the future
- feel anger at the injustice of institutional prejudice and people's worldview.

They may need:

- an adult to listen to them and be curious about their feelings and experiences
- to experience an adult defend them and vindicate them if they have been treated unfairly
- to reflect on any experiences and what change can be facilitated that brings justice to those who have been misunderstood or judged unfairly
- to have opportunities that others may have, with apologies if they have ever been overlooked or misunderstood
- to have an input into any changes that need to be achieved in the trauma-informed system and culture
- kindness, empathy, compassion and time to reflect and be heard
- an older mentor who has navigated their way through the injustice and can give ideas for how to flourish.

## The criminal justice system

Many children and families who have faced trauma, such as abuse or violence, are invited to go through the criminal justice system to seek justice and to try and stop others being hurt by the same person. Sadly, the far too common response from children is that the system is not child centred and can be significantly traumatizing. The system needs to be updated in many ways, and while changes are beginning to be made, they are not applied equally across the nations. The current statistics demonstrate that most people who go through this system for crimes such as abuse or harassment rarely get the justice they sought. However, there are exciting signs of hope as new models are being created to enable children's voices and stories to be heard without them feeling further traumatized. In Scotland, the new Bairns Hoose model for children is pioneering a better way for children to access the justice system and feel supported appropriately along the way.

The child may feel:

- terrified of being judged or misunderstood by adults in authority
- terrified of being accused of lying when they are telling the truth
- terrified of having to repeat their story and remember details that they would rather forget
- exhausted by the meetings and questions and different adults who don't always seem to communicate well with each other
- desperate to move on and forget the whole traumatic event and let someone else fight for them instead.

They may need:

- empathy and compassion for what they are having to go through
- the space to explore and express emotions about the injustice of what they are having to do as a victim of crime
- the ability to find ways to soothe themselves when they are being asked questions or being interviewed
- an adult to continually explain what will happen next, what they need to do and why, so that they feel supported on the journey towards justice and less powerless
- ways to express different difficult emotions that they may feel, such as anxiety, distress, anger, rage and terror
- to hear stories from other children who have navigated their way through the system.

## Other organizational trauma experiences

There are so many other traumatic experiences, such as *gang violence, sexual exploitation and trafficking*, that cannot be explored in so few lines when the injustice causes such destruction to the lives of those who are impacted. These experiences often involve sexual trauma, physical trauma and psychological trauma, which are explored in Section 2. The additional trauma theme is one of betrayal, loss and relationship or 'interpersonal' trauma, where they have been hurt by those they trusted. This can take time to process and the coping mechanisms that are used to survive such a Type III trauma need to be slowly recognized, understood and validated before the child can stop using them.

'Organized abuse occurs when one or more abusers collude to abuse one, or a number of unrelated children…[and] can include darker themes of torture, degradation and extreme cruelty' (Schofield, 2021, p.12). This form of abuse tends to include ritual, high levels of organization and deliberate conditioning of the mind for the purpose of lifelong mind control; it is 'built on lies and manipulation of attachment needs' (Miller, 2012, p.xvii). This is more common than most of society would like to believe. It is beyond the remit of this book to cover this area as it deserves, but a good starting point might include Alison Miller's books, some written for survivors and others for professionals, most recently *Demystifying Mind Control and Ritual Abuse* (2024).

There is spiritual and religious abuse, where leaders render those who attend powerless to challenge, defend, discuss or reflect on what is being taught, suggested or practised. A person's desire to belong and be accepted can be challenged, threatened or controlled. The leaders abuse their power to secretly, overtly or subtly manipulate, control or use people who trust them, with fear, ghosting and mockery. Leaders should care for the people they lead and never misuse their position.

The child may feel:

- a sense of injustice, terror and confusion
- stuck and powerless, with a fear of their story not being believed
- many emotions that need space to be expressed, seen, heard and validated
- shame that they became victims of any of these organizational trauma experiences
- the need to be listened to and shown empathy and kindness.

They may need:

- support from caring and empathetic adults
- validation for the depth of their distressing feelings
- time for them to explore how they feel, what they are worried about and what they need, with the same committed supportive adult
- some help to dream about the future after the trauma has stopped and they can begin to heal and enjoy pursuing their talents and interests
- time to heal rather than a rushed, short-term support package

- the areas of the child's life that have been impacted by the trauma to be intentionally recovered, as explored in Section 2.

## Conclusion

There are many different themes within organizational trauma. One is around the environments that are not trauma informed or human centred, and so the people who are interacting with that environment feel small, powerless and not valued. Organizational trauma can be devastating because the powerlessness of trauma can be increased as the person feels unable to 'fight' against a person *and* 'a system'. The experience of fighting for justice when injustice has been normalized can feel pointless, and many people feel exhausted and unable to keep fighting unless they join with others who share the same passion to see justice. Corruption and evil do exist, and living with the reality that some people have been given power and are using it to harm others can be difficult to acknowledge and accept. It is important to not be alone but reach out to others to find empathy, compassion and care and to fuel each other's passion to keep fighting in the space that you are in until you feel as if you've done what you can. Sometimes it's necessary to step down and hand the baton to someone else to fight so that you can recover and learn to enjoy life.

## Further reading

- *A Treasure Box for Creating Trauma-Informed Organizations: A Ready-to-Use Resource for Trauma, Adversity, and Culturally Informed, Infused and Responsive Systems* (Therapeutic Treasures Collection) by Karen Treisman (2021). Jessica Kingsley Publishers.

# CHAPTER 23

# Emotional Neglect

Emotional neglect can look like a child who:

- doesn't have enough nurture, warmth, emotional connection and kindness
- doesn't feel celebrated, known, seen and heard
- has enough food and toys but is left alone or in front of screens for hours a day
- feels abandoned and alone
- feels primarily present to help and serve other family members
- is made to be independent too quickly
- is not treated with the appropriate change of boundaries in relationship because they now need peers more than their parents
- is looked after by multiple different adults to whom they are not emotionally connected
- is only celebrated for what they achieve and not for who they are
- is withdrawn and has no adults who look forward to them being present.

Here is a quote from Chapter 1 of my book *The Simple Guide to Emotional Neglect*, which explores how to recover from emotional neglect:

Emotional neglect and unmet emotional needs seem to be experiences that people can't always easily understand, comprehend or empathize with, even though we know that the primary experience for the baby and child of not having an emotionally connected adult is being terrified, powerless and overwhelmed.

There is a whole continuum of emotional neglect. It starts on one end with the distress and stress that a child experiences when they have unmet emotional needs. On the other end of the continuum, where the child is caused deep distress by the unmet emotional needs and the consequences of that distress are then seen in behaviours, emotions and trauma symptoms, emotional neglect can be a criminal offence. Child emotional neglect at the most severe end of the continuum is also defined as child cruelty and therefore child abuse, due to the level of deprivation. It is vital that we don't refuse to notice what we see to 'avoid judgement' when we suspect that a child is in a situation such as this, but instead it is vital to immediately involve child protection services (police and social workers) who need to help the child urgently. Often in situations where neglect is the issue, adults around them can unintentionally collude with the neglect and can become apathetic to the obvious needs of the child (Wolock & Horowitz 1984). We recognize that while 'removal' from those settings is not in any way the whole answer, it can be an important factor for the child's safety and can reduce the further impact of developmental trauma. Further along the emotional neglect continuum would be the desperate lack of emotional connection which can feel like a matter of life and death to a child, although they would rarely be able to put that into words. At the other end of the continuum the child has unmet emotional needs that lead to coping mechanisms that can be interruptive to their healthy development.

Emotional neglect could be explained as the ongoing lack of emotional responsiveness to the child, where the parent doesn't notice what the child may be feeling, doesn't try to help them explore what may be going on and doesn't validate their experiences enough. The child feels that their feelings are consistently ignored, unvalidated and disregarded by their parent.

Emotional neglect leads to emotional trauma, which is a word used interchangeably with psychological trauma, to differentiate it from physical traumatic injury that requires surgeons, doctors and medics to facilitate healing.

We know that as humans we seem to find that bruises elicit less empathy than wounds with blood, even if the bruise is life-threatening, and emotional trauma can often feel like that.

'I lied and told the teacher my friend's mum had died of cancer, because I couldn't answer her question about why I was always sighing in class and struggling to concentrate. I didn't know what or if anything was

wrong with me. I guess I just knew I was sad and felt overwhelmed.'
Sophie, aged 16, who grew up with emotional neglect. (de Thierry, 2023,
pp.16–18)

# CHAPTER 24

# Collective Trauma

Here is a short quote from the beginning of my book *The Simple Guide to Collective Trauma*, which explores the impact of collective trauma:

> While the collective trauma is shared, people will have varied experiences of it and will respond to these experiences differently, depending on their own personal backgrounds and current context.
>
> This book will explore the impact of collective trauma on children and young people but also on adults, because the impact on the adults has a direct effect on the younger generation. Sometimes I will refer to the impact on 'people', because it is similar for both children and adults.
>
> Collective trauma can impact us all, but not all of us are traumatized by events and experiences which are traumatic for others. Some people may experience stress or a crisis, but it doesn't have to cause long-term traumatic impact. Usually, the degree of traumatic impact of any terrifying experience is connected to the child's ability to find comfort and reassurance from a safe and known adult, both in the immediate aftermath of the experience and then as a safe place to further explore the experience over time. (de Thierry 2021, p.17)

Collective trauma can be caused by events such as:

- war
- natural disasters such as tsunamis, fires, floods etc.
- mass shootings or public violence
- genocides
- pandemics
- terrorist attacks
- economic disasters

- any other one-off traumatic event which is witnessed by a collective of people
- a continual traumatic repeated event, which is ongoing, with ongoing impact and shock. (de Thierry 2021, p.18)

The book explores the different experiences, different symptoms and ways to help facilitate recovery.

# NAVIGATING THE SYSTEM AND THE TRAUMA RECOVERY FOCUSED MODEL®

# CHAPTER 25

# Navigating the Current System of Help

Many of you who are reading this may have asked for help from either your doctor, school, a mental health team or a specialist provision, and you are now waiting for someone to be available to support you in helping the child move away from a difficult space in their life, where the trauma is impacting them.

To help you feel less powerless as you wait for help, I want to equip you to make sure that the help the child eventually receives is what is needed rather than yet another short-term provision that only seems to put the brakes on the struggles and doesn't offer long-term solutions. Too many children are eventually offered some short-term help, but when the planned weeks of sessions have ended, things seem to go back to how they were before or become worse due to another feeling of loss. This keeps many families in the mental health system for many years, and that shouldn't be the case.

Let's explore the maze of help offered so that you can make sure that the treatment suggested for your child is the best option for them.

## Different offers of help or therapeutic modalities

Many professionals believe that their specific method/modality/training is the one way to heal someone who has been traumatized. Sadly, that is rarely the case. The training, modality and skills that are needed to help facilitate recovery in each area of the child's life that has been impacted by trauma require a trauma recovery model that uses a combination of different tools and knowledge. Most of us have had to do multiple different trainings to be able to help children recover from trauma.

As you wait for help to be available, you may not be aware that the qualifications and experience of staff on most mental health teams can vary in incredible ways, and access to that information can be difficult. Although it can often seem that any help is better than no help at all, that is not necessarily true with trauma, because it can take a long time for a child to learn to trust an adult, and if that adult is then unable to facilitate the needed recovery, the disappointment can lead to the child taking even longer the next time to trust another adult or not wanting to trust anyone for a very long time. In fact, after a few times of 'trying the help offered' the child can often be heard to say that they don't want to risk another professional again. Sometimes they can then be viewed as 'hard to engage', but we know that they are probably rightfully nervous and sensitive about trusting yet another adult who promises to know how to help them recover from trauma but seems to get stuck or annoyed at their lack of progress. For a traumatized child, it can be deeply detrimental to their long-term recovery to have different professionals who seem unable to confidently help them through to positive recovery, and this can escalate the trauma and increase the symptoms. Therefore, it is always advisable to ask some questions from the professional who is available to help the child:

- What qualifications does the person have?
- How many years of experience do they have?
- How were they trained?
- What specialist area have they focused on?
- What books or trauma theorists have been influential for them?
- What are their aims?

I would also suggest that the child meets the adult and is empowered to decide if they feel that they could engage with the process. This introduction process is vital for long-term recovery and is sometimes rushed due to the desperation to get any help.

## Trauma training for professionals

Many newly qualified professionals are taught to work in a certain way to achieve a certain result, and sadly many will use words such as 'to help them process their trauma' while they are not actually specifically trained to assess the trauma impact and create a treatment plan that is going to effectively do so. Currently, I am not aware of many courses in any nation that equip a professional over several years of study to fully help the child navigate through a one-to-two-year journey of trauma recovery with each and every area of trauma impact addressed in this book. I have facilitated a ten-day certificate and have trained psychotherapists, counsellors, mental health nurses, occupational therapists, social workers, paediatricians, doctors, nurses, health visitors, headteachers, teachers, learning support assistants, police, music, art and play therapists, educational psychologists and many others who have not been familiar with the content of my Trauma Recovery Focused Model®.

Many professionals are trying to learn about trauma but there are increasing numbers of courses that are available for them, and it's important for them and you to have evidence of the course trainer and their experience of leading families through to trauma recovery. Each trainer should have data to evidence that they have experience of being in this role, and you should be able to read something that they have written to evidence this in context, such as a case study. Otherwise, they are just training from material they have been given from a course they have attended, and the knowledge becomes diluted with more and more people facilitating the information, which becomes second or third hand.

*If you needed a life-changing surgical operation, such as a C-section, would you rather the surgeon who performs your operation in the hospital had been taught by surgeons who had years of experience or would you be comfortable with them being trained by someone who themselves had a C-section and had been to a training on it from a surgeon over a few days but had no medical training or qualifications?*

As the qualifying course usually does not equip the professional to be fully trained specifically to help facilitate trauma recovery, the evidence will be in their work data and/or their writing and people's evaluations of their practice.

There are many modalities that do help a person recover from trauma, but most are aimed at only one aspect of the trauma impact, and so the child often ends up having to re-enter a waiting list for further help a few years later because some symptoms were not targeted by that professional.

## Relationships

Trauma happens in the context of relationships. The trauma experience is either the direct actions of someone who hurts the child or the inaccessibility, unavailability or not quite sufficiently attuned caregiving of the child's primary caregiver to provide comfort and reassurance in the face of distress or pain. As a parent of four, I am more than aware that it is can sometimes be or feel almost impossible to continually provide to the children all the emotionally available, emotionally connected and attuned caregiving that is needed for the healthy development of children. Sometimes things happen in life, and we can experience our own trauma, which can interrupt our ability to be as present as we would like for our children, and so we are not blaming or shaming anyone. What is recognized, however, is that the harm has taken place in the context of relationship, and recovery from trauma must therefore involve longer-term relationship experiences that are positive and healing. That is often the starting point for most therapeutic methods that are aimed at helping trauma recovery. For a child to be able to go through the process of recovery and healing, they need to have trust in the adult with whom they are sharing the depths of their terror and challenges. That is not a quick process. The longer the child has been without an adult whom they feel they can trust, who is emotionally available for them to express all the range of emotions without filter and help them process what's happened to them, the longer it will take for them to learn to trust an adult now.

## Parent blame

Please be aware that we are not blaming the parent if they were not able to be emotionally available to the child, because we don't know what was going on for them. They may have been victim to the same abuse or neglect, they may have been preoccupied with another crisis or trauma where they were trying to protect the child and were unaware that ironically and horrifically something else was harming their child. It could be that the parent was focusing on providing food and a home and that was all they could do with the limited resources they had, but meanwhile the child felt alone, isolated and abandoned. It could be that the parent was unwell and was trying with everything they had to be emotionally available, but the child had decided that they didn't want to harm their deeply loved parent further and so pretended they were fine, while harbouring deep feelings of confusion and hurt that they pushed down to protect their relationship. Relationships are complex, and we can all try our best with the knowledge and resources that we have been given at the time, so we need to create atmospheres where there is no shame or judgement.

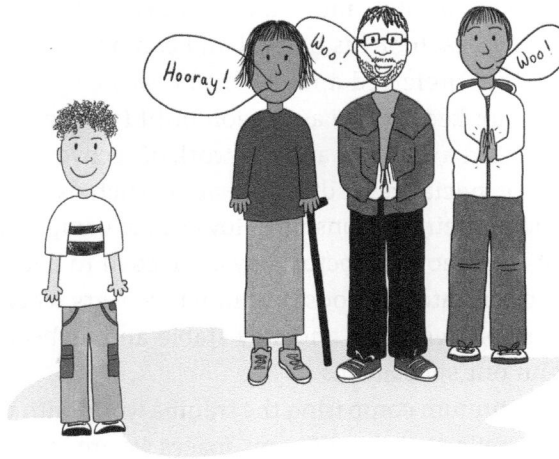

The first barrier to recovery and healing that needs to be overcome is the child being able to build healthy, therapeutic relationships, preferably with several adults. The more long term these can be, the better outcomes for recovery because further loss and feelings of rejection can be avoided.

## Different professionals and their qualifications: The continuum of role

Trauma recovery is different from the management of behaviour and symptoms. When we focus on managing, we are working to stop the unhelpful symptoms and behaviours that can often be interruptive to the child and those around them. Management is a different focus from recovery. I believe that recovery is possible, using a different lens through which to view symptoms and behaviours, which are ways of coping with the deep feelings of distress that are causing turmoil. A recovery-focused lens is one where we recognize that as the distress is lessened, the symptoms and behaviours change. Therefore, we focus on helping the child to process, make sense of and externalize the distress in ways that naturally decrease the power it has on their lives. This then decreases the interruptive symptoms and behaviours.

To facilitate trauma recovery, it takes a team, in the same way that to facilitate a child's recovery from severe sickness also requires a team who have different roles within the recovery journey. Each person in the team is vital, and while the roles and training for the roles are different, each one is helpful and can be necessary. When I was giving birth, I preferred a midwife who was a specialist in that field and I was not keen to see a surgeon until I needed one. Ideally, people do not need a surgeon and the work of recovery can be done with those who specialize in different areas such as emotions, the body, the mind or their relationships. However, in complex trauma, an equivalent of a surgeon or doctor may be needed to help with some of the more complicated periods of trauma recovery where it is hard for the child to process pain and stay stable and feel safe. We need each other and our specialisms.

Here is a continuum comparing the trauma world with the medical work to help us reflect on the different spaces we are in:

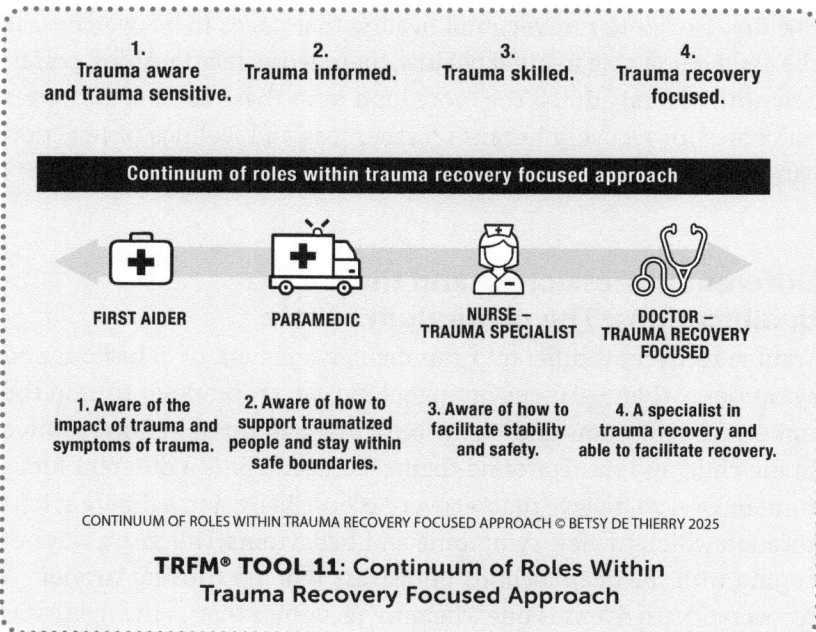

| 1. Trauma aware and trauma sensitive. | 2. Trauma informed. | 3. Trauma skilled. | 4. Trauma recovery focused. |
|---|---|---|---|

**Continuum of roles within trauma recovery focused approach**

| FIRST AIDER | PARAMEDIC | NURSE – TRAUMA SPECIALIST | DOCTOR – TRAUMA RECOVERY FOCUSED |
|---|---|---|---|
| 1. Aware of the impact of trauma and symptoms of trauma. | 2. Aware of how to support traumatized people and stay within safe boundaries. | 3. Aware of how to facilitate stability and safety. | 4. A specialist in trauma recovery and able to facilitate recovery. |

CONTINUUM OF ROLES WITHIN TRAUMA RECOVERY FOCUSED APPROACH © BETSY DE THIERRY 2025

**TRFM® TOOL 11**: Continuum of Roles Within Trauma Recovery Focused Approach

We recognize how helpful it is to have first aiders at a sports match or a school, and in the same way it would be ideal to have all adults learn to be trauma first aiders. A trauma first aider can help calm and support a person who is feeling frightened or shocked, without judgement or panic. They may have done a mental health first-aid course or an introduction to trauma training. The trauma-informed 'paramedic' is an adult who has confidence to check that cultures, policies, approaches and systems all ensure that all adults are guided by 'four assumptions, known as the "Four R's". These are the Realization about trauma and how it can affect people and groups, Recognizing the signs of trauma, having a system which can Respond to trauma, and Resisting re-traumatization' (Substance Abuse and Mental Health Services Administration, 2014). In my Trauma Recovery Focused Model®, the first aider is the mentor or parent, the paramedic is the professional who can work to change cultures and inspire policies and practice, and the 'nurse' is the psychotherapist or psychologist who can clinically assess the trauma symptoms and history and create a trauma treatment plan to enable the child to recover from what has happened to them. The 'doctor' is similarly qualified but more experienced than the professional, taught the nurse to conduct the assessments and can carry out the complex subconscious processing in partnership with the 'nurse', who offers longer-term support. Ideally, the 'first aider', 'paramedic', 'nurse' and 'doctor' work together to support the child over a year or more, with the 'first aider' or 'paramedic' being available and accessible throughout the week, the 'nurse' being the consistent adult for weekly sessions, and the 'doctor' coming in for some specific specialist moments.

## A brief summary of who does what in the children's mental health world

It is important that you have some idea who you are asking for help from. All of these professionals are hardworking, caring people who have committed their lives to helping others. Therefore, we should be grateful that they have all spent so many years training! This is a very short overview of where they may fit within a trauma recovery lens.

## Doctors and paediatricians

These are highly trained, over approximately seven challenging years, to understand in depth how the body and brain work and what to do with different illnesses or accidents that harm the body. They are always highly intelligent, and general medical doctors (GPs in the UK) have had to spend years and years in different areas of medical specialism in order to then become a local doctor available for people to book an appointment with.

They are trained to understand medication and would be able to listen to symptoms of mental health challenges and interpret how those fit with different diagnoses as presented in the *Diagnostic Statistical Manual of Mental Health Disorders*, and then what medication could help the symptoms decrease. They are, however, not trained yet (2024) to understand the impact of trauma on various different presentations unless they have chosen to study it as continuing professional development. This means that recovery from trauma is rarely the lens that they are viewing the symptoms through.

'Paediatricians are incredibly passionate about children thriving and fulfilling their potential. We have the joy of seeing children recover from ill-health, but we have to support children and families through extraordinary pain and grief too. While our training equips us well to diagnose and respond to many health needs, training in psychological trauma and the amazing things children's brains and bodies do to navigate fear and survive remains inadequate and patchy, often dependent on gutsy local champions who can see that the dominant medical model of child mental health understanding and symptom management is failing children and families, and who are trying to build better pathways to trauma recovery. All doctors would benefit from understanding our shared human responses to adversity and trauma through this trauma recovery lens. Not only would we be better placed to serve our patients and advocate for national systems that help children and families thrive – serious matters of health and justice – but we would be better equipped to care for ourselves and each other too in this challenging world.' *Dr L.C. Wood, forensic paediatrician*

## Educational psychologists

'Educational psychologists (EPs) have either a Masters in Educational Psychology, or a doctorate in educational psychology (mandatory since 2006). Some EPs are also qualified teachers. All practising psychologists are registered with the Health and Care Professions Council (HCPC) and must meet their standards of conduct, proficiency and ongoing professional development. EPs also practise in line with professional codes of ethics, such as those of the British Psychological Society.

'EPs aim to improve the learning and overall wellbeing of children. They work with children, parents, school staff and other professionals in order to support a child's ability to succeed. EPs work in many contexts, including the local authority, multi-academy trusts, private EP services and so on. Every child is unique, and EPs try to unpick what might be going on for them, in order to generate solutions to help learning and wellbeing. An EP assessment may involve: consultation with parents/teachers, questionnaires, observation of the child at school, gaining the child's views, and/or cognitive/learning assessments. Outcomes are recorded in reports which outline what has been found and the subsequent support required to meet the child's needs. EPs do not generally diagnose neurodevelopmental conditions, but they may be a part of this process. Many EPs have not had specific training in trauma, but will have an in-depth understanding of attachment and child development theory. There are very few EPs who have completed training in trauma recovery.' *Dr Sarah Gothard, educational psychologist*

## Children and Adolescent Mental Health Service (CAMHS)

This is the UK group of professionals who are the first place that children usually get referred for help. Every location has a CAMHS team, and the professionals on that team can change due to staff movement, so the regional teams vary in what they offer. Each staff member has a very varying level of training, which is worth enquiring about before the child meets with them to explore access to support. The CAMHS team often encompasses a psychiatrist, psychologists, psychotherapists, counsellors, occupational therapists, mental health nurses, mental health first aiders, social workers, and trainees of all of those qualifying courses. It is important to know who your child is being offered an appointment with. Some regions will have sub-projects to offer specialized support, some will be trained to understand trauma recovery and occasionally there may be a specialized team within CAMHS that is trauma recovery focused, but each region varies considerably.

## Social work professionals

Here is a thought from a social worker on her training and the application of this book:

'There are a broad range of lenses in which social workers are trained to consider and enhance their critical reflection, assess needs, review care plans and advocate and navigate systems to support individuals across all stages of life. However, being trauma recovery focused is a vital lens that is not yet taught as a core component within training programmes – but if it were, would radically transform social workers' practice and therefore the lives of the individuals and communities they are passionate to support! Embedding trauma recovery focused training into every social worker's qualification would fundamentally shift the long-term care of individuals, communities and this nation and is the ethical approach we so urgently need in our generation.' *Jess Nash, social worker and play therapist*

## Occupational therapists

'Occupational therapists (OTs) help people with their daily activities or 'occupations'. OTs may do this by working on a particular movement or skill, suggesting changes to the environment, providing equipment or developing strategies to help the individual participate.

'As an OT, trauma recovery did not form part of our core training. In fact, in an OT context, when people talk about 'trauma', they are generally referring to serious physical injuries resulting from an accident. All the training I have completed about trauma recovery has been after qualifying, with OT-specific courses only being available relatively recently.

'The role of the OT in trauma recovery is definitely developing and becoming more evidence based, so it is exciting to see things changing, but there is still a long way to go!' *Vanessa Battle, occupational therapist*

## Psychotherapists, psychologists and art, music, play, drama and dance therapists

These professionals belong to a regulating board which has checked their qualifications and holds ethics and values of professional practice that they have to adhere to. You can ask which regulating board the therapist is a member of. All of them should have clinical supervision monthly or more frequently, where they discuss the children and adults they are helping, anonymously, with a qualified clinician who has experience working with similar children or families. Both their membership of a regulating board and their clinical supervisor help them stay safe and help you know that others have checked and are checking their practice continually.

## Holding a doctorate or PhD in a mental health subject

I started a PhD and then had my fourth child instead, deferred for a year, but then my supervisor had left that university and so I deferred for longer. The process of further study is an academic one rather than an ongoing experience of being in the position of facilitating trauma recovery. Therefore, I would argue that having this level of qualification enables the professional to have a very high level of expertise in one narrow subject matter that they have researched. This is usually immensely helpful in shaping the world of psychology but does not usually increase their interpersonal skills in facilitating trauma recovery for more complex cases.

# CHAPTER 26

# My Trauma Recovery Focused Model®

This book is an overview of the Trauma Recovery Focused Model® that I originally created for the Trauma Recovery Centres (TRC®s) that I founded in 2011 to use to facilitate trauma recovery with the children, young people, parents, carers and schools who work with us.. It is not a tick list, but an overall sense of progression towards healing and recovery, in a wiggly way!

It is important to recognize that many professionals are doing an incredible job in providing crisis recovery, where they can offer skilled support to those who have experienced trauma, especially when they are first needing help to recover from the shock of the traumatic experience. These professionals are able to offer a supportive, emotionally connecting relationship that can facilitate the recovery from crisis to a sense of re-found stability and hope. This is not how I would define trauma recovery because that is a longer and more complex process that is built on the foundation of safety and stability, but requires additional skills that include the ability to process trauma from the unconscious and reduce the need for any hidden or obvious coping mechanisms, which I would describe as symptoms of surviving trauma. Judith Herman (1998) suggests that recovery:

> unfolds in three stages. The central task of the first stage is the establishment of safety. The central task of the second stage is remembrance and mourning. The central task of the third stage is reconnection with ordinary life. Treatment must be appropriate to the patient's stage of recovery. A form of therapy that may be useful at one stage may be of little use or even harmful to the same patient at another stage.

My model is a different from hers but similar in the aims of recovery. Most trauma models begin with the establishment of safety because until that happens, nothing more can be done to facilitate healing.

This is a brief overview and the skills and tools are explored in my training programme.

## The Trauma Recovery Focused Model® (TRFM®)
### TRFM® First foundation stage: STEPS TOWARDS HOPE AND SAFETY – CRISIS RECOVERY

*Parent/carer or therapeutic mentor is able to lead this without a therapist if they have been trained to use these tools.*

- Beginning to build positive, healthy attachment relationships that co-regulate and facilitate emotional safety.
- Building and working towards the child's physical safety and environmental safety.
- Assessing the child's trauma history and symptoms using the trauma continuum (de Thierry, 2015).

### TRFM® Second foundation stage: SAFETY, STABILITY AND REGULATION

*Parent/carer or therapeutic mentor is able to lead this stage without a therapist if they have been trained to use these tools.*

- Emotional safety is beginning to be developed and strengthened through the key relationships and those facilitating positive experiences.
- The nervous system becomes understood, and the child can notice when they are outside their Window of Tolerance.
- The child is able to use different emotional regulation tools that bring comfort, soothing, calm and energy to guide them close to or into the Window of Tolerance with their key adults, and they begin to be able to use them on their own too.
- The child has a sense of hope for recovery and wants to be on the journey.
- The child begins to use knowledge that they have been taught about their brain and emotions when speaking about

experiences and events of the week to evidence their understanding of psychoeducation.

- Shame is beginning to reduce as psychoeducation empowers the
child to understand themselves and what is going on!
- A basic VIP or daisy map (de Thierry, 2015) is explored by the
child with reflection regarding any dissociation that may be
present.
- Emotions become validated, unstuck, expressed, understood
and noticed.
- Relationships become safe and secure, and warning signs are
acknowledged.
- Habits become healthier, and that is reflected in their sleep, diet,
exercise and hobbies.

## TRFM® Third stage of trauma recovery:
## SYMPTOM ACCEPTANCE AND REDUCTION,
## AND TRAUMA PROCESSING

*From here it would be ideal for them to have a therapist who first learns
and practises with them the tools from the foundation stages before beginning to assess the trauma symptoms and working on the body, emotions,
mind and relationships.*

- There is an emerging stability in their life in terms of home,
school and attachment relationships.
- They can increasingly recognize their own trauma symptoms
and explore what purpose they serve.
- Thinking patterns become less out of control and negative
beliefs can be noted and challenged.
- The body becomes known, cared for and listened to, and begins
to be understood.
- They begin to feel safer in their body as they understand what
the body is communicating and why.
- Any internal dissociative system is mapped and explored.
- They can begin to process some more simple trauma memories
which interrupt their life – slowly and carefully.
- They can grieve over that which has been lost and feel a range
of other emotions.

## TRFM® Fourth stage of trauma recovery:
## INTEGRATIVE NARRATIVE AND RECOVERY

- They can begin to be able to use words to describe the trauma experiences and how they feel about them.
- They begin to recognize the need for and the way that trauma memories need to be processed and be keen to get on with that when the new memories arise.
- Triggers are understood, predicted and no longer limit their life.
- The child can be present in the moment instead of disconnecting and dissociating to numbness.
- The subconscious memories and coping mechanisms become understood.
- The child's identity begins to strengthen in ways that are not connected to the trauma.
- They grow in skills that were otherwise not able to flourish due to the trauma.
- Memories become conscious and less invasive, and they continue to process trauma memories as any surface.
- The daisy becomes less chaotic and disintegrated, less out of control, more organized, and it has fewer 'petals' as integration is facilitated.
- Identity becomes less chaotic and disintegrated and more integrated and confident.
- A sense of predictability and integrity of behaviour and relationships has been formed from the integration process.

Once the first stage has been the focus and seems to be developing well and the child has some sense of a relational safe base, there should be some sense of moving through the stages sequentially. There is also a realization that humans don't move on from one stage to another without repeating all the stages, with the general sense of an overall progression towards increasing safety, stabilization, knowledge of the trauma, symptoms and coping mechanisms, and an increased sense of healing, integration and restoration.

The TRFM® aims can be summarized by the word REBUILD:

## THE REBUILD MODEL SUMMARY

**R** ebuilding lives

**E** ducating around trauma

**B** uilding positive healing relationships

**U** ndoing the impact of shame

**I** nvestigating the subconscious

**L** ook at the whole story of your survival

**D** are to live fully!

THE REBUILD MODEL SUMMARY © BETSY DE THIERRY 2025

**TRFM® TOOL 12: The Rebuild Model Summary**

As explored in Section 1, trauma recovery needs to start with building a foundation of safety and stability, which can take some time. This is essential before trauma can be processed, and also throughout the journey.

## My TRFM® approach

In this specific trauma recovery treatment model that I created, each child has a creative psychotherapist and a therapeutic mentor, and they build positive attachment relationships with both. The therapist is the one who leads the work, which involves continually completing the clinical assessments; ongoing building of the healthy foundations with psychoeducation and emotional co-regulation; facilitating activities that enable the nervous system to become more 'organized'; facilitation of the slow mapping of the subconscious systems; while also facilitating the processing of body memories, trauma memories and the forming of the trauma integrative narrative. The therapeutic mentor can help with the consolidation weeks when they need to occur and can be another friendly person if the therapist is unwell so that there is consistency in weekly sessions. The therapeutic mentor can also facilitate emotional regulation, psychoeducation work and sensory activities that the therapist has prepared for them to do.

Our parenting support team use my *Parenting the Traumatised Child* curriculum to lead the parenting groups, where parents and carers are able to feel supported and emotionally held while they learn, discuss, reflect and work out how to help the child begin to heal. The children can begin access to the centre by joining a creative therapeutic programme and can also revisit that space where they have found safety and healing. I believe we need spaces that enable children to have long-term attachment to places as well as individuals. This pioneering model has data that evidences that the child almost always recovers from trauma. Other organizations can partner with the TRFM® and be licensed to follow it, with the training and resources available.

## Hope on the wiggly journey

Trauma recovery can be a challenging road to travel but it can be increasingly positive as glimmers of hope and change shine in the darkness of the wiggly road. This book aims to provide some comforting streetlights to help you navigate some of the main areas of the confusing journey. As you keep travelling with hope and compassion as your strengths and companions, slowly the darkness becomes less murky, and clarity increases about what has happened and what impact that has had. The child begins to come back to life as the weight of the trauma they are carrying is lessened, enabling them to begin to demonstrate who they are with a new confidence.

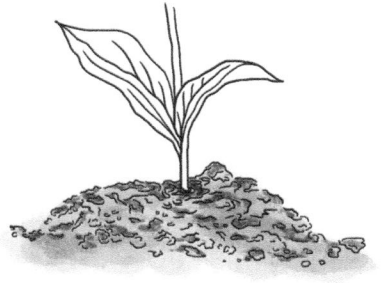

As you grow in confidence about the different terrains on the recovery journey and what tools you need to navigate them, I hope you will find that trauma recovery is possible and that emotions, body memories, beliefs and negative thoughts, internal dissociative systems and relationships can transform from being fragmented and full of turmoil and pain to being filled with hope.

As we all work hard to see young lives changed and recover from trauma, it can then change the trajectory of a generation. The invisible scars of trauma no longer cause devastating turmoil and pain, and they can bring hope to others who are starting their journey. There should be no shame for the scars that are left behind, as they are signs of a painful road travelled with courage, where others can follow on after us, with more signposts that we have left behind.

Well done for changing lives and helping children and young people find hope and safety!

# References

Arain, M., Haque, M., Johal, L., Mathur, P. *et al.* (2013). Maturation of the adolescent brain. *Neuropsychiatric Disease and Treatment*, 9, 449–461. doi: 10.2147/NDT.S39776.

Ayres, A.J. (1989). *Sensory Integration and Praxis Tests*. Los Angeles, CA: Western Psychological Services.

Badenoch, K. (2015). *Silent Suffering: Supporting the Male Survivors of Sexual Assault*. GLA Conservatives, 15 November. https://glaconservatives.co.uk/_files/ugd/047866_67bcc6def2ab4314b69b3148a0df8a00.pdf.

Boyle, K. (2010). Introduction. In K. Boyle (ed.), *Everyday Pornography*. London: Routledge.

Brooks, S.K., Webster, R.K., Smith, L.E., Woodland, L. *et al.* (2020). The psychological impact of quarantine and how to reduce it: Rapid review of the evidence. *The Lancet*, 395, 912–920. doi: 10.2139/ssrn.3532534.

Brown, B. (2015). *Rising Strong*. London: Vermillon Publishing.

Brown, B. (2021). *Atlas of The Heart: Mapping Meaningful Connection and the Language of Human Experience*. London: Penguin Random House.

Brown, B. (2024). *The Practice of Story Stewardship*. 5 December 2021 (Accessed June 2024).

Brown, F. (2014). The healing power of play: Therapeutic work with chronically neglected and abused children. *Children* (Basel, Switzerland), 1(3), 474–488. https://doi.org/10.3390/children1030474.

Burgess, A.A. & Holmstrom, L.L. (1974). Rape trauma syndrome. *American Journal of Psychiatry*, 131 (1974), 981–986.

Cantor, P., Osher, D., Berg, J., Steyer, L. & Rose, T. (2018). Malleability, plasticity, and individuality: How children learn and develop in context. *Applied Developmental Science*, 23(4), 307–337. https://doi.org/10.1080/10888691.2017.1398649.

Carr, E. (2014). *Parental Apologies: A Catalyst to Optimal Parenting*. Conference paper. doi: 10.13140/2.1.1253.2482.

CBC Radio. (2022). Are we mislabeling our trauma? Why Dr. Gabor Maté believes we need to change the way we think about pain. www.cbc.ca/radio/

thenextchapter/are-we-mislabeling-our-trauma-why-dr-gabor-mat%C3%A9-believes-we-need-to-change-the-way-we-think-about-pain-1.6661540.

Cénat, J.M. (2023). Complex racial trauma: Evidence, theory, assessment, and treatment. *Perspectives on Psychological Science: A Journal of the Association for Psychological Science*, 18(3), 675–687. https://doi.org/10.1177/17456916221120428.

Colman, A.M. (ed.) (2008). *A Dictionary of Psychology (third edition)*. Oxford: Oxford University Press.

Coy, M., Kelly, L., Elvines, F., Garner, M. & Kanyeredzi, A. (2013). '*Sex without consent, I suppose that is rape': How young people in England understand sexual consent.* London: Office of the Children's Commissioner.

Coyne, I. & Conlan, J. (2007). Children's and young people's views of hospitalization: 'It's a scary place'. *Journal of Children's and Young People's Nursing*, 1(1), 16–21. doi: 10.12968/jcyn.2007.1.1.23302.

Cozolino, L. (2006). *The Neuroscience of Human Relationships: Attachment and the Developing Social Brain (Norton Series on Interpersonal Neurobiology)*. New York, NY: W.W. Norton & Company.

Crown Prosecution Service. (2023). Controlling or Coercive Behaviour in an Intimate or Family Relationship. www.cps.gov.uk/legal-guidance/controlling-or-coercive-behaviour-intimate-or-family-relationship.

Crummy, A. & Downey, C. (2022). The impact of childhood trauma on children's wellbeing and adult behavior. *European Journal of Trauma & Dissociation*, 6(1), 100237. www.sciencedirect.com/science/article/pii/S2468749921000375.

Davies, P. & Martin, M. (2008). Children's emotional security in the interparental relationship. *Current Directions in Psychological Science*, 17, 269–274. doi: 10.1111/j.1467-8721.2008.00588.x.

D'Elia, D., Carpinelli, L. & Savarese, G. (2022). Post-traumatic play in child victims of adverse childhood experiences: A pilot study with the MCAST-Manchester Child Attachment Story Task and the Coding of PTCP Markers. *Children (Basel, Switzerland)*, 9(12). https://doi.org/10.3390/children9121991.

de Thierry, B. (2015). *Teaching the Child on the Trauma Continuum*. London: Grosvenor Publishing.

de Thierry, B. (2016). *The Simple Guide to Child Trauma*. London: Jessica Kingsley Publishers.

de Thierry, B. (2017). *The Simple Guide to Sensitive Boys*. London: Jessica Kingsley Publishers.

de Thierry, B. (2018). *The Simple Guide to Understanding Shame in Children*. London: Jessica Kingsley Publishers.

de Thierry, B. (2019). *The Simple Guide to Attachment Difficulties*. London: Jessica Kingsley Publishers.

de Thierry, B. (2020). *The Simple Guide to Complex Trauma and Dissociation*. London: Jessica Kingsley Publishers.

de Thierry, B. (2021). *The Simple Guide to Collective Trauma*. London: Jessica Kingsley Publishers.

de Thierry, B. (2023). *The Simple Guide to Emotional Neglect*. London: Jessica Kingsley Publishers

Dvir, Y., Ford, J.D., Hill, M. & Frazier, J.A. (2014). Childhood maltreatment, emotional dysregulation, and psychiatric comorbidities. *Harvard Review of Psychiatry*, 22(3), 149–161. https://doi.org/10.1097/HRP.0000000000000014.

Ede, G. (2024). *Change Your Diet, Change Your Mind*. London: Hodder and Stoughton.

Federal Bureau of Investigation. (2017). UCR Program. Crime in the US: Rape. https://ucr.fbi.gov/crime-in-the-u.s/2017/crime-in-the-u.s.-2017/topic-pages/rape.

Fisher, J. (2017). *Healing the Fragmented Selves of Trauma Survivors*. London: Routledge.

Fosha, D., Siegel D. & Solomon , M. (2009). *The Healing Power of Emotion: Affective Neuroscience, Development & Clinical Practice*. New York, NY: W.W Norton & Company.

Flood, M. (2009). The harms of pornography exposure among children and young people. *Child Abuse Review*, 18(6) 384–400.

Gamache Martin, C., Van Ryzin, M.J. & Dishion, T.J. (2016). Profiles of childhood trauma: Betrayal, frequency, and psychological distress in late adolescence. *Psychological Trauma: Theory, Research, Practice, and Policy*, 8(2), 206–213. https://doi.org/10.1037/tra0000095.

Garcia, G. (2017). *Listening to My Body: A guide to helping kids understand the connection between their sensations (what the heck are those?) and feelings so that they can get better at figuring out what they need*. Skinned Knee Publishing.

Gerhardt, S. (2004). *Why Love Matters*. Hove, East Sussex: Brunner-Routledge.

Gilbert, P. (2015). Self-Disgust, Self-Hatred, and Compassion-Focused Therapy. In P.A. Powell, P.G. Overton & J. Simpson (eds), *The Revolting Self: Perspectives on the Psychological, Social, and Clinical Implications of Self-Directed Disgust* (pp.223–242). London: Karnac Books.

Gomez, A. & Hosey, J. (2025). *The Handbook for Child Complex Trauma and Dissociation: Theory, Research, and Clinical Applications*. London: Routledge.

Gomez-Perales, N. (2015). *Attachment-Focused Trauma Treatment for Children and Adolescents: Phase-Oriented Strategies for Addressing Complex Trauma Disorders*. New York, NY: Routledge.

Gross, Y. (2020). Erikson's Stages of Psychosocial Development. In B.J. Carducci & C.S. Nave (eds), *The Wiley Encyclopedia of Personality and Individual Differences: Models and Theories Volume 1* (pp.179–184). Hoboken, NJ: John Wiley & Sons.

Hanson, E. (2020). *What is the impact of pornography on young people? A research briefing for educators*. London: PSHE Association.

Hart, S.N., Brassard, M.R. & Karlson, H.C. (1996). Psychological Maltreatment. In J.N. Briere, L.A. Berliner, J. Bulkley, C.A. Jenny & T.A. Reid (eds), *The APSAC Handbook on Child Maltreatment*. Thousand Oaks, CA: Sage.

Herman, J.L. (1998). Recovery from psychological trauma. *Psychiatry and Clinical Neurosciences*, 52(S1), S98–S103. https://doi.org/10.1046/j.1440-1819.1998.0520s5S145.x.

Herman, J. (2022). *Trauma and Recovery; The Aftermath of Violence from Domestic Abuse to Political Terror*. (Original work published 1992.) New York, NY: Basic Books.

Horvath, M.A.H, Alys, L., Massey, K., Pina, A., Scally, M. & Adler, J. (2013). *'Basically...porn is everywhere': A Rapid Evidence Assessment on the Effects that Access and Exposure to Pornography has on Children and Young People*. London: Office of Children's Commissioner.

Hughes, D. & Golding, K.S. (2012). *Creating Loving Attachments: Parenting with PACE to Nurture Confidence and Security in the Troubled Child*. London: Jessica Kingsley Publishers.

Hyland, P., Murphy, J., Shevlin, M., Vallières, F. *et al.* (2017). Variation in post-traumatic response: The role of trauma type in predicting ICD-11 PTSD and CPTSD symptoms. *Social Psychiatry and Psychiatric Epidemiology*, *52*(6), 727–736. 10.1007/s00127-017-1350-8.

Iram Rizvi, S.F. & Najam, N. (2014). Parental Psychological Abuse toward children and mental health problems in adolescence. *Pakistan Journal of Medical Sciences*, 30(2), 256–260.

Iyendo Jnr, T. & Alibaba, H. (2014). Enhancing the hospital healing environment through art and day-lighting for user's therapeutic process. *International Journal of Arts and Commerce*, 3, 111–119.

Jung, C. (1973). *Memories, Dreams, Reflections*. New York, NY: Random House.

Kalisch, L., Lawrence, K., Baud, J., Spencer-Smith, M. & Ure, A. (2023). Therapeutic supports for neurodiverse children who have experienced interpersonal trauma: A scoping review. *Review Journal of Autism and Developmental Disorders*, 1–23. 10.1007/s40489-023-00363-9.

Kessler, R.C., McLaughlin, K.A., Green, J.G., Gruber, M.J. *et al.* (2010). Childhood adversities and adult psychopathology in the WHO World Mental Health Surveys. *The British Journal of Psychiatry*, 197(5), 378–385. https://doi.org/10.1192/bjp.bp.110.080499.

Klaassen, M.J. & Peter, J. (2015). Gender (in)equality in internet pornography: A content analysis of popular pornographic internet videos. *The Journal of Sex Research*, 52(7), 721–735.

Laliotis, D., Philadelphia, M., Oren, P., Shapiro, E. *et al.* (2021). What Is EMDR therapy? Past, present, and future directions. *Journal of EMDR Practice and Research.*, 15. doi: 10.1891/EMDR-D-21-00029.

Larrinaga-Undabarrena, A., Río, X., Sáez, I., Angulo-Garay, G. *et al.* (2023). Physical activity levels and sleep in schoolchildren (6-17) with and without school sport. *International Journal of Environmental Research and Public Health*, 20(2), 1263. https://doi.org/10.3390/ijerph20021263.

Levine, P. (1997). *Waking The Tiger: Healing Trauma*. Berkeley, CA: North Atlantic Books.

Levine, P. & Kline, M. (2017). *Trauma Through a Child's Eyes*. Berkeley, CA: North Atlantic Books.

Lerwick, J.L. (2016). Minimizing pediatric healthcare-induced anxiety and trauma. *World Journal of Clinical Pediatrics*, 5(2), 143–150. https://doi.org/10.5409/wjcp.v5.i2.143.

Li, X. (2023). Emotion understanding, expression, and regulation in early childhood. *Journal of Education, Humanities and Social Sciences*, 15, 25–30. doi: 10.54097/ehss.v15i.9055.

Li, Y., Xia, X., Meng, F. & Zhang, C. (2022). The association of physical fitness with mental health in children: A serial multiple mediation model. *Current Psychology*, 41(10), 7280–7289. https://doi.org/10.1007/s12144-020-01327-6.

Loades, M.E., Chatburn, E., Higson-Sweeney, N., Reynolds, S. *et al.* (2020). Rapid systematic review: The impact of social isolation and loneliness on the mental health of children and adolescents in the context of COVID-19. *Journal of the American Academy of Child & Adolescent Psychiatry*, 59(11), 1218–1239. doi: 10.1016/j.jaac.2020.05.009.

López-Zerón, G. & Blow, A. (2015). The role of relationships and families in healing from trauma. *Journal of Family Therapy*, 39. doi: 10.1111/1467-6427.12089.

Malamuth, N. (2001). Pornography. In N.J. Smelser & P.B. Baltes (eds), *International Encyclopedia of Social and Behavioral Sciences*, 17, 11816–11821.

Masten, C.L., Guyer, A.E., Hodgdon, H.B., McClure, E.B. *et al.* (2008). Recognition of facial emotions among maltreated children with high rates of post-traumatic stress disorder. *Child Abuse & Neglect*, 32(1), 139–153. doi: 10.1016/j.chiabu.2007.09.006.

Maté, G. (1999). Scattered Minds. The Origins and Healing of Attention Deficit Disorder. London: Penguin Random House.

McLeod, D. & Flood, S. (2018). *Coercive Control: Impacts on Children and Young People in the Family Environment*. Dartington: Research in Practice.

Mearns, D. & Cooper, M. (2005). *Working at Relational Depth in Counselling and Psychotherapy*. London: Sage.

Merriam-Webster Dictionary (2024). Terror. www.merriam-webster.com/dictionary/terror.

Mezey, G.C. & Taylor, P. J. (1988). Psychological reactions of women who have been raped: A descriptive and comparative study. *The British Journal of Psychiatry*, 152, 330–339. https://doi.org/10.1192/bjp.152.3.330.

Miller, A. (2012). *Healing the Unimaginable: Treating Ritual Abuse and Mind Control*. London: Routledge.

Music, G. (2019). *Nurturing Children: From Trauma to Growth Using Attachment Theory, Psychoanalysis and Neurobiology*. London. Routledge.

Myers, C.S. (1915). A contribution to the study of shell shock: Being an account of three cases of loss of memory, vision, smell, and taste, admitted into the Duchess of Westminster's War Hospital, Le Touquet. *The Lancet*, 185(4772), 316–320. https://doi.org/10.1016/S0140-6736(00)52916-X.

National Child Traumatic Stress Network. (n.d.). Trauma types. Sexual Abuse. www.nctsn.org/what-is-child-trauma/trauma-types/sexual-abuse.

National Child Traumatic Stress Network (2008). Child Trauma Toolkit for Educators [PDF file]. www.nctsn.org/resources/child-trauma-toolkit-educators.

NHS England. (2022). *Supporting Male Victims/Survivors Accessing a Sexual Assault Referral Centre Good Practice Guide*. www.england.nhs.uk/wp-content/uploads/2022/02/B1313_Supporting-male-victims-survivors-accessing-a-sexual-assault-referral-centre-good-practice-guide-Februar.pdf.

Nicholson, J. (2020). *The Power of Play Power of Play for Addressing Trauma in the Early Years*. www.researchgate.net/publication/341273839_The_The_Power_of_Play_Power_of_Play_for_Addressing_Trauma_in_the_Early_Years.

NSPCC. (2024). Domestic abuse. www.nspcc.org.uk/what-is-child-abuse/types-of-abuse/domestic-abuse/#what.

Panchal, U., Salazar De Pablo, G., Franco, M., Moreno, C. *et al.* (2021). The impact of COVID-19 lockdown on child and adolescent mental health: Systematic review. *European Child & Adolescent Psychiatry*, 1–27. 10.1007/s00787-021-01856-w.

Perry, B.D. (2014). The Neurosequential Model of Therapeutics: Application of a developmentally sensitive and neurobiology-informed approach to clinical problem solving in maltreated children. In K. Brandt, B.D. Perry, S. Seligman & E. Tronick (eds), *Infant and Early Childhood Mental Health: Core Concepts and Clinical Practice* (pp.21–53). Washington, DC: American Psychiatric Publishing.

Perry, B.D. & Szalavitz, M. (2010). *Born for Love: Why Empathy is Essential—and Endangered*. New York, NY: William Morrow.

Perry, B.D. & Winfrey, O. (2021). *What Happened to You?* London: Flatiron Books.

Phippen, A. (2012). *Sexting: An Exploration of Practices, Attitudes and Influences*. London: NSPCC.

Porges, S.W. (1993). The infant's sixth sense: Awareness and regulation of bodily processes. *Zero to Three: Bulletin of the National Center for Clinical Infant Programs*, 14, 12–16.

Porges, S. (2011). *The Polyvagal Theory: Neurophysiological Foundations of Emotions, Attachment, Communication, and Self-Regulation*. New York, NY: W.W. Norton & Company.

Porges, S. (2017). *The Pocket Guide to the Polyvagal Theory*. New York, NY: W.W. Norton & Company.

Putnam, F.W. (1997). *Dissociation in Children and Adolescents: A Developmental Perspective*. New York, NY: Guilford Press.

Rees, C. (2007). Childhood attachment. *British Journal of General Practice*, 57(544), 920–922. doi: 10.3399/096016407782317955.

Safran, J.D. & Muran, J.C. (2000). Resolving therapeutic alliance ruptures: Diversity and integration. *Journal of Clinical Psychology*, 56(2), 233–243.

Saracho, O. (2021). Theories of child development and their impact on early childhood education and care. *Early Childhood Education Journal*, 51, 15–30. https://doi.org/10.1007/s10643-021-01271-5.

Schlote, S. (2023). History of the term 'appeasement': A response to Bailey *et al.* (2023). *European Journal of Psychotraumatology*, 14(2), 2183005. https://doi.org/10.1080/20008066.2023.2183005.

Schofield, L. (2021). Understanding Dissociative Identity Disorder: A Guidebook for Survivors and Practitioners. London: Routledge.

Shetty, J. (2023). 'Gabor Maté & Jay Shetty on Understanding Trauma.' Jay Shetty blog, 3 October 2023. www.jayshetty.me/blog/gabor-mate-and-jay-shetty-on-understanding-trauma.

Siegel, D. (2012). *The Whole Brained Child: 12 Proven Strategies to Nurture Your Child's Developing Mind*. London: Robinson Publishing.

Silberg, J. (2012). *The Child Survivor: Healing Developmental Trauma and Dissociation*. London: Routledge.

Spodek, B. & Saracho, O.N. (1999). The relationship between theories of child development and the early childhood curriculum. *Early Child Development and Care*, 152(1), 1–15. https://doi.org/10.1080/0300443991520101.

Substance Abuse and Mental Health Services Administration (SAMHSA). (2014). *SAMHSA's Concept of Trauma and Guidance for a Trauma-Informed Approach.* Rockville, MD: Substance Abuse and Mental Health Services Administration.

Thomas, J.C. & Kopel, J. (2023). Male victims of sexual assault: A review of the literature. *Behavioral Sciences* (Basel, Switzerland), 13(4), 304. https://doi.org/10.3390/bs13040304.

United Nations. (1989). Convention on the Rights of the Child. Treaty Series, 1577, 3. Chicago, IL.

van der Kolk, B.A. (2014). *The Body Keeps the Score: Brain, Mind, and Body in the Healing of Trauma*. New York, NY: Viking.

Vythilingam, M., Heim, C., Newport, J., Miller, A.H. *et al.* (2002). Childhood trauma associated with smaller hippocampal volume in women with major depression. *The American Journal of Psychiatry*, 159(12), 2072–2080. https://doi.org/10.1176/appi.ajp.159.12.2072.

Waters, F. (2016). *Healing the Fractured Child: Diagnosis and Treatment of Youth with Dissociation*. New York, NY: Springer Publishing.

Watkins, J.G. & Watkins, H.H. (1979) The Theory and Practice of Egostate Therapy. In H. Grayson (ed.), *Short Term Approaches to Psychotherapy*. New York, NY: Human Sciences Press.

Weindl, D. & Lueger-Schuster, B. (2018). Coming to terms with oneself: A mixed methods approach to perceived self-esteem of adult survivors of childhood maltreatment in foster care settings. *BMC Psychology*, 6(1), 1–12. doi: 10.1186/s40359-018-0259-7.

Wieland, S. (2011). *Dissociation in Traumatised Children and Adolescents*. New York, NY: Routledge.

Winnicott, D.W. (1953). Transitional object and transitional phenomena. *International Journal of Psychoanalysis*, 34, 89–97.

Winston's Wish (2020). *Do children grieve differently to adults?* https://winston-swish.org/do-children-grieve-differently.

Wolke, D. & Lereya, S.T. (2015). Long-term effects of bullying. *Archives of Disease in Childhood*, 100(9), 879–885. https://doi.org/10.1136/archdischild-2014-306667.

Yang, F.N., Xie, W. & Wang, Z. (2022). Effects of sleep duration on neurocognitive development in early adolescents in the USA: A propensity score matched, longitudinal, observational study. *Lancet Child Adolescent Health*, 6(10), 705–712. doi: 10.1016/S2352-4642(22)00188-2.

# Subject Index

# Author Index